BREATHE
AS YOU ARE

BREATHE
AS YOU ARE

Harmonious Breathing for Everyone

FABIO ANDRICO

SHANG SHUNG PUBLICATIONS

DISCLAIMER: The content of this book is intended for general information purposes only. The guidance provided here is not meant to replace medical advice. Always consult your physician before implementing any of the suggestions in this book. Any application of the material presented herein is at the reader's discretion and is his or her sole responsibility.

Art direction and cover design: Mandarava Bricaire and Richard De Angelis
Book design and illustrations: Richard De Angelis
Draft layout: Francesco Festa
Photography: Marc Benera, Mandarava Bricaire, Kamal Rodríguez, Adrien Pilet, and Vince Li Wen Tai
Portrait of Fabio Andrico: Alison Sam
Editors: Susan Schwarz and Vicki Sidley

Copyright © 2017 Shang Shung Foundation
Published by Shang Shung Publications,
an imprint of the Shang Shung Foundation
Merigar
58031 Arcidosso (GR)
http://shop.shangshungfoundation.com

ISBN 978-88-7834-159-3

CONTENTS

APPENDIX 1 | WARM-UPS 124

PREFACE

We come into life with our first breath. We are alive because we breathe. The reality is that the way we breathe is easily one of the most important factors influencing our physical, mental, and energetic well-being.

Unfortunately, rather than breathing in an open and natural way, most people breathe with tension. If tension in the breathing becomes a habit, it throws our energy out of balance and ultimately can lead to stress, anxiety, and poor health.

So why not try to breathe well? Why not do something to discover, experientially, what it's like to breathe without tension? Instead of allowing our respiration to become a source of unbalanced energy and ultimately poor health, it is in our own power to develop a breathing pattern that can regenerate our vital force, give us good energy, promote health and well-being, and help us overcome tension and stress.

Often, the only thing standing in our way is that we lack the knowledge and the tools to understand and learn how. We do not know how to experience and reshape our breathing patterns to a way that is more complete, more natural, and of greater benefit.

My primary purpose for writing this book is to share a series of simple exercises for discovering and experiencing the movement of respiration in a more complete and natural way. The exercises explained here form the basis of Harmonious Breathing, a system I have developed to help people from all walks of life and with very different physical conditions develop a respiratory pattern of complete breathing, where the inhalations fluidly combine an abdominal, an intercostal, and a thoracic phase, and the exhalations consist of an equally fluid sequence in the reverse order.

By doing the Harmonious Breathing exercises presented here, you teach your body to breathe completely, and by doing them consistently, the quality of complete breathing integrates with your normal breathing pattern. On a mechanical level, consistent complete breathing improves the tone of the diaphragm, one of the most important muscles in your body, and that, in turn, increases your lung capacity and favorably affects the quality of your respiration.

This is not a book about yoga. And yet, yoga, particularly Yantra Yoga, a Tibetan practice first brought to the West by Dzogchen master Chögyal Namkhai Norbu, has had the most formative influence on my understanding of breathing.

Four decades of dedicated yoga practice – including more than thirty years as a yoga teacher (mainly of Yantra Yoga) – have led me to recognize and experience that breathing is one of the most central, fundamental aspects of the discipline, not least of everyone's life. Time and again, I saw that many people, regardless how much or how little interest they may have in seriously pursuing a practice like yoga, simply want to learn how to breathe well. In time, drawing on my past experience, I began to teach workshops just on breathing.

Since we all have to breathe – whether we are young or old, thin or not, flexible or not, practice yoga or not – this book is designed to be useful for everyone, for anyone who wants to rediscover the importance and the beauty of breathing in a fluid, smooth, harmonious, and natural way. The aim is to breathe in a way that is as tension-free as possible.

What is important is to be able to have a concrete experience, feeling that the benefit of what we practiced is becoming something tangible, something that will extend beyond the moment of practice and into our everyday life.

The Harmonious Breathing exercises will make you more aware of your body, and you will come to know it better. You will experience more energy, life force, vitality, and strength. At the core of these qualities is the harmonious condition of joyful breathing – the beautiful seed of gentle and tension-free strength.

It's not about creating something new. It's about rediscovering something that was always there, but was covered by tension. Something that can make our life better.

This book is structured much like a Harmonious Breathing workshop, starting with an overview of what defines complete breathing, then taking you through a series of exercises that will help you understand complete breathing experientially and give you the tools to start developing a healthy, harmonious breathing pattern. None of the exercises in this book require familiarity with yoga or other types of bodywork, and you will easily be able to put together a routine that suits your time, circumstances, and condition. Additionally, a number of suggested routines are offered in appendix 2.

Since any session ideally begins with at least a few warm-ups, appendix 1 contains a large selection of warm-up exercises to choose from. Warming up is a good way to prepare for breathwork and also improves your overall flexibility and health.

Both the core Harmonious Breathing exercises and the warm-ups are also identified by level (easy, moderate, and challenging), and a separate index lists each exercise according to those three categories.

In this book, we will not be exploring in depth the various techniques and characteristics of holding the breath, as this topic is extensively explained and applied in Yantra Yoga, for example, where it forms an integral part, the core, of the practice.

The differences between various schools and systems are not covered in this book. Nor, with the exception of a brief overview in the appendix, will we be looking at anatomy and physiology. My intention is not to produce an academic study, but to provide an understanding of a fluid, natural way to breathe, to offer a practical guidebook based on four decades of experience.

In addition to working with the inhalation and exhalation, another important aspect of breathing practices in yoga – if not the most important one – is the retention of the breath. Holding the breath in a controlled manner has innumerable benefits, but since it is such a powerful tool, it should be learned in the context of a system that can guarantee that it is done in the proper way.

Here, we will use only a simple, and yet effective, retention of the breath, and only in very few exercises. We will apply a gentle suspension of the breathing following the natural tendency of the spontaneous movement of our respiration to briefly retain the breath after inhalation and after exhalation. A pause after an inhalation is what we call "open hold." A pause after an exhalation is called "empty hold."

Retaining the breath in this way – smoothly and gently – has a soothing, relaxing, and harmonizing effect, and helps deepen the already great benefits of conscious, fluid respiration: Tension-free respiration, not energy free. Full of energy, but relaxed energy. Focused and free of obstacles, free of forceful struggle. Free to flow. Free to unfold the natural vigor of life.

ACKNOWLEDGMENTS

So many people played a role in the process that led me to write this book that it is impossible to name them all. The people I learned from or who helped me along the way include writers, researchers, and scientists who conducted serious experiments on the effects of breathing. Then there are all the people who worked with me directly on the production of this book. Each and every one of them is in my mind and my heart, and the ones I know personally are very much aware of the place they have in my life.

Thank you to you all.

More than anything I am deeply grateful to my teacher Chögyal Namkhai Norbu for the immense gift of his profound wisdom and compassion.

INTRODUCTION

BREATH IS LIFE

Breathing is the door to our energy, the bridge that connects the mind and the body. If our body and energy are relaxed, our mind, too, can have little or no tension and finally relax. Conscious, mindful breathing, mindful movements of our body, and a correctly and naturally aligned position allow our inner harmony to manifest.

Practicing some simple breathing exercises can help us discover or, better said, rediscover a more natural flow of our respiration, a different, more harmonious dimension.

The subject of breathing has been widely covered, both from the medical perspective (in particular in terms of anatomy and physiology), and from the perspective of yoga, which includes the science of breath among its practices. However, the various schools of yoga and other systems of breath-based exercises differ in their points of view regarding the actual workings of the physiology of breathing, and not all schools and systems consider breathing to be the most important aspect. In Yantra Yoga the quality of the breath is crucial, a central feature of the practice. More specifically, it guides us to experientially discover and develop various ways of breathing and in so doing unlock the patterns that prevent us from breathing to our full potential.

Not everyone wants to or can practice yoga. Not everyone has the time, capacity, predisposition, and interest to do so. But everyone breathes. So why not learn how to do it well?

This concrete knowledge conveyed by Yantra Yoga is the source and inspiration of the step-by-step system I designed to help everyone – regardless of body type, age, capacity, or prior experience – develop a complete breathing pattern. I call it Harmonious Breathing.

Despite all variances, one common principle is shared among all styles and methods of breathing practice: Breathing is life. Mind and breathing are interconnected.

If you are agitated, you will have constricted, agitated respiration. If, on the contrary, you are calm and emotionally tension free, your breathing will be calmer and smoother. By coordinating your breathing, you will coordinate your energy and relax your mind. You will experience a more aware, calm, clear, and vital mind, and a new energy in your life. You will also develop a healthier body.

As Chögyal Namkhai Norbu explains, "Our breathing is connected to and conditioned by our mind, by emotions. When we are nervous we breathe with nervousness. When happy, we breathe with happiness. When worried, we breathe with worry, because breathing is influenced by the mind, is conditioned by the mind, and the mind is often confused, distracted, and tense. In Yantra Yoga we say that breathing is like a blind horse and the mind like a lame rider. The lame rider can ride the horse and so the horse can be controlled. Everything is interdependent. So, if we are in control of our breathing or have some control over the mind, everything becomes easier. For this reason first of all we have to stabilize our respiration."

First and foremost, we need to understand the importance of breathing in a fluid, smooth, harmonious, and natural way.

Also, in nearly all yoga exercises, we are taught to inhale and exhale mainly through the nostrils, through the filter of the nose. It is better to always inhale and exhale through the nostrils outside of practice as well.

We can take short breaths or long ones. A breath can be fast and vigorous or long, smooth, and subtle. We have different circumstances in our life, different states of mind. The breath is linked to all the movements of our life: the movements of our mind, our energy, and our body. So of course our breathing changes in response to circumstances – and it needs to. But when the inner core, the soul of our breathing, is tension free and in a naturally relaxed condition, an inner harmony will always be there.

Because our body and energy are conditioned by tensions, by our mind and our emotions, we generally do not use our full breathing potential. We breathe in a shallow and limited way. Our breath is often fragmented, tense, and unharmonious. It does not flow. Also, some people have a tendency to overbreathe, even when at rest. Learning how to relax and coordinate our breathing can help with all these problems.

In response to stress, we tend to develop shallow breathing patterns that set off a chain of consequences that begin with inefficient oxygen/carbon dioxide exchange and a progressive degeneration of our vital organs and go on to affect our entire being. The vital cycle of inhaling and exhaling becomes a vicious circle in which we are increasingly incapable of handling stress, easily fall into anxiety and depression, and develop systemic imbalances.

When we breathe deeply, the diaphragm gently massages our organs and stimulates blood flow, promoting health, longevity, and well-being. Relaxed breathing relaxes our state of mind and fosters constructive coping mechanisms. It's not for nothing that the first advice for responding to challenges is often "just breathe."

Our mental and physical health is related to the condition of our energy. Knowing how to apply deep, relaxed, and complete breathing is the first milestone on the way to achieving true and lasting well-being.

This does not mean, however, that the goal is to apply a pattern of deep, complete breathing at all times and in all circumstances. Rather, as yoga therapist Leslie Kaminoff puts it, by "exploring the full potential of our breathing mechanisms" we can "uncover and dismantle habitual patterns that obstruct normal function."

THE ENERGETIC DIMENSION OF BREATHING

In our ordinary, busy lives it is difficult to have a concrete experience and direct knowledge of the energetic dimension of the body, much less to know how to be able to control it or influence it. We can, however, learn to control our breathing. In fact, by coordinating the inflow and outflow of breath we are able to balance specific functions of the *prana*. The circulation of *prana* in our body determines the condition of our energy. It can be controlled, balanced, and harmonized.

Tibetan medicine and Ayurveda (the medical system of India) are founded on the knowledge of what we might call "the anatomy of energy," an important part of which is the theory of the five elements: earth, water, fire, air, and space. The five elements, according to Tibetan medicine and Ayurveda, are the base, the foundation, of our physical, material condition, and are the essence underlying all. Each element has its own function, nature, and quality. Sickness arises when the five elements are imbalanced, when one or more of the elements are either in excess, deficient, or disturbed. By developing a healthy breathing pattern we can balance and strengthen the condition of the five elements and as a consequence overcome many physical, energetic, and mental problems.

According to both Tibetan medicine and Ayurveda, the five elements give rise to three distinct energies that form the basis for the functioning of the human body. When these three energies – called wind, bile, and phlegm in the Tibetan system – are in balance and in proper relationship to each other, we have a perfect state of health. If they are imbalanced or in excess or deficient or abnormal in their interaction with each other, we experience disorders and diseases.

In order to be healthy we need to bring these elements and energies back into balance and keep them all in harmony. In fact, harmonizing our breathing patterns is a key factor in restoring natural balance.

If we want to be wholesome, if we want our well-being to be stable, we should work with our breathing. But all is interconnected, interdependent. We also need to work with our body to help relax tensions and allow a natural coordination of the breathing. This will coordinate our energy and help relax the mind.

If, in turn, the mind is less tense, more relaxed, the breathing will become more calm and the body less tense, less blocked, more flexible. The result is a powerful synergy between our body, energy, and mind.

We need to discover and understand our energy, the movement of our energy. It is important not to be afraid of our energy manifesting, flowing. Instead of obstructing it or blocking it, we can embrace it with harmony and joy. By learning how to cultivate our energy, we can experience the beauty and power of our inner, subtle strength manifesting. We can change the perception of our life, harmonize the movement of life. Breathing better is the best place to start.

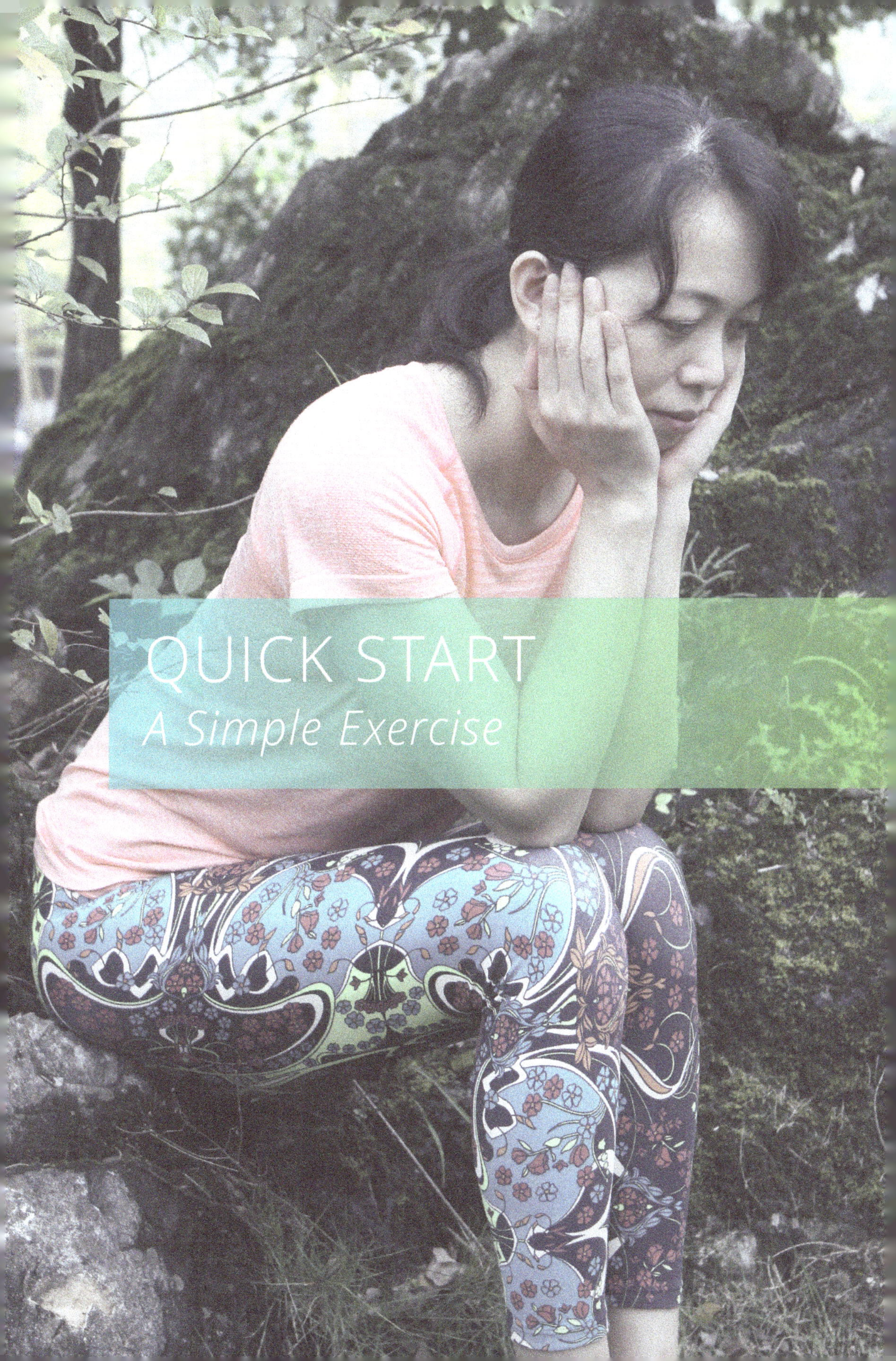

QUICK START

A Simple Exercise

QUICK START: A SIMPLE EXERCISE

J ust to give you an idea of what Harmonious Breathing is all about, here's a simple, three-part exercise that you can do on the floor or sitting on a chair.

The purpose of this exercise is to give you a concrete, immediate experience of smoother, more open, and relaxed breathing. It will help you discover a different dimension of respiration and lead you to understand on a direct, visceral level how Harmonious Breathing works.

FLOOR VERSION   CHAIR VERSION

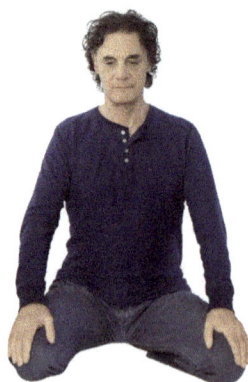

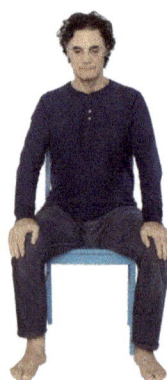

Starting position

FLOOR VERSION

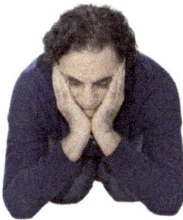

Kneel with your back straight, knees together or loosely apart, hands on or above the knees, and one foot placed on top of or next to the other. If needed, you can place a pillow under your buttocks to make the position more comfortable.

CHAIR VERSION

Sit near the edge of a chair with your back straight and hands on or above your knees, at first keeping the knees parallel or loosely apart.

For a few rounds of breath, just observe your breathing, without trying to do anything with it. Just be aware of inhaling and exhaling. Be sure to give yourself time to notice the quality of your breathing pattern. Every now and then take a deep inhalation, then go back to unmodified breathing.

FLOOR VERSION

CHAIR VERSION

First position

Now bend forward, place your elbows on the floor in front of your knees, and rest your chin in your hands. If this position of the hands is not comfortable for your neck, you can lower your head slightly and rest your cheeks in your hands.

Now place your elbows on the thighs just above your knees (be sure to find a point where it is comfortable) and rest your chin or cheeks in your hands.

Breathe, alternating calm, relaxed respiration with a more active, intentional expansion on the inhalation – for just one or two minutes.

Second position

Then open your knees and move the elbows as far apart as comfortable, with yours hands still holding your chin.

Then, seated in the same position, open your knees wider and as before rest your chin in your cupped hands.

Breathe, alternating calm, relaxed respiration with a more active, intentional expansion on the inhalation – for just one or two minutes.

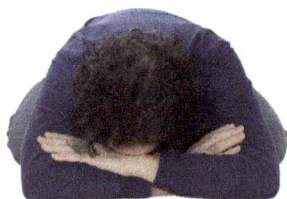

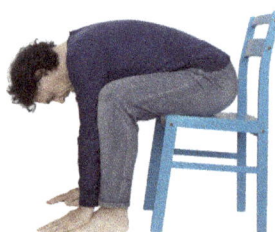

Third position

Finally, without changing the position of your legs, cross your arms in front of you and place your forehead on them.

Finally, keeping the knees wide open, bend forward and down, placing your hands on or near your feet and relaxing your head. Alternatively, simply cross your arms (keeping the elbows just above the knees), and rest your forehead on your arms.

Breathe, alternating calm, relaxed respiration with a more active, intentional expansion on the inhalation – for just one or two minutes.

FLOOR VERSION   CHAIR VERSION

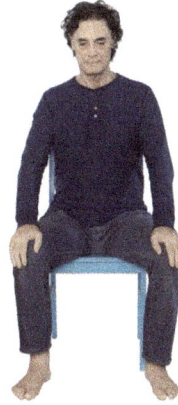

Conclusion

To end, rise up into a sitting position with your back straight.

Without wanting to do anything in particular with your breathing, just notice how it is. Observe and experience the flow of the breath, its quality.

Notice if there is any difference in the breathing now from the way it was before applying these exercises.

This sequence can also be done as a short and simple routine to center yourself on your breathing, to be mindful of the smooth flow of your respiration. You can do it whenever you feel the desire or the need to let go, and effortlessly experience the pleasure of being present and relaxed. You can do it at the office when you are overloaded. It will help you relax and center in just a few minutes.

Now that you've had a little taste of a different quality of breathing, you're ready to start learning a skill that will bring you long-lasting benefit.

PART 1 |

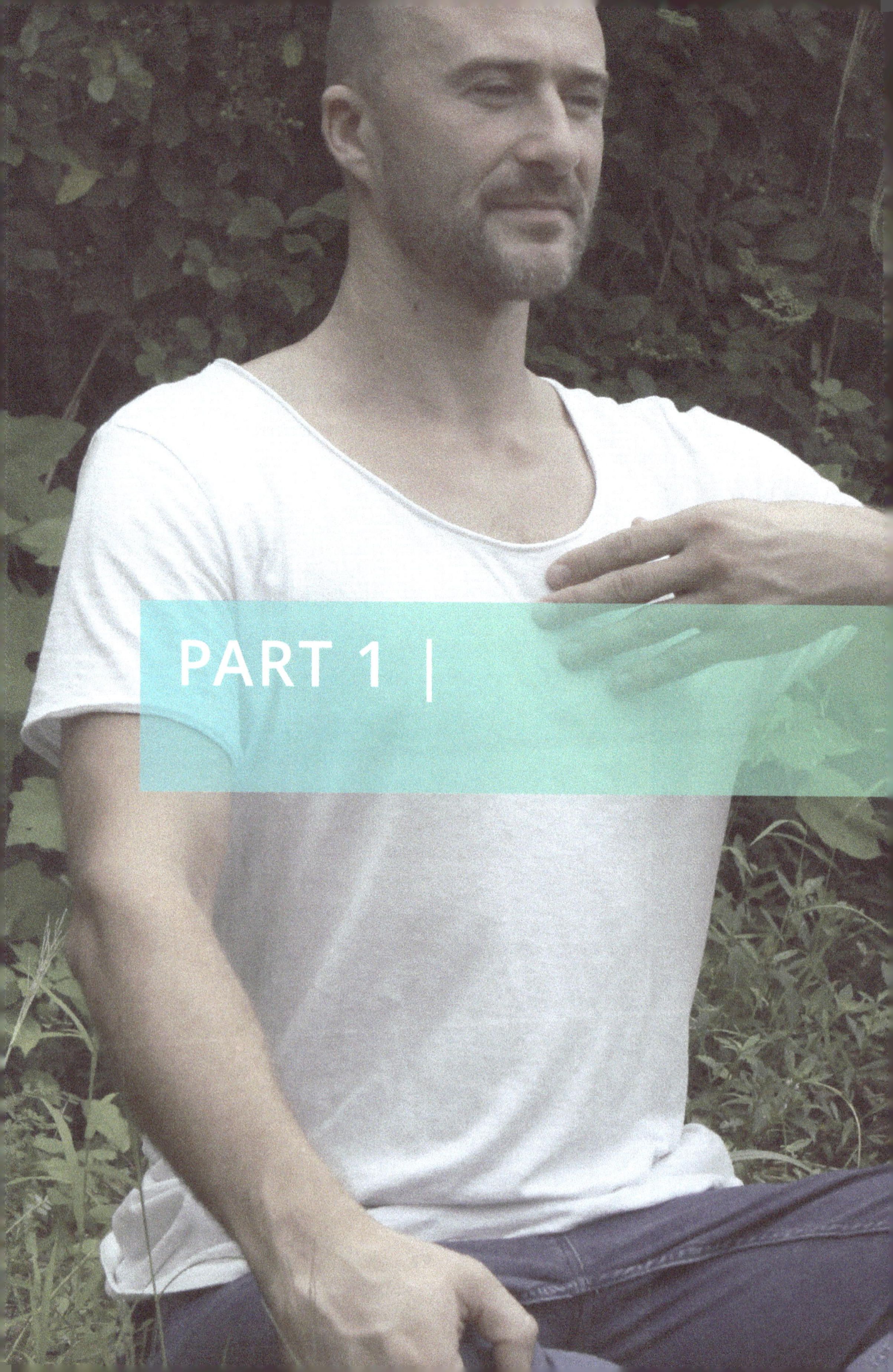

COMPLETE BREATHING IN THEORY

COMPLETE BREATHING IN THEORY

A BRIEF OVERVIEW

Complete breathing is an ideal and complete respiratory pattern in which both inhalation and exhalation fluidly combine an abdominal, an intercostal, and a thoracic phase. Occasionally, the third phase is further subdivided into a chest phase and an upper chest phase, making four in all. In addition, each phase can be augmented with a dorsal expansion. Harmonious Breathing is a simple and effective method that teaches us how to develop a complete breathing pattern and make it a constant part of our lives. It is a method of learning by doing, of exploring and discovering.

Because the division into four phases is more effective for the learning process, Harmonious Breathing makes use of the four-phase approach along with dorsal expansion.

The best place to start is to make sure you are breathing in a fluid, smooth, harmonious, and natural way through the nostrils.

Nearly all types of yoga teach us to inhale and exhale mainly through the nostrils, through the filter of the nose. This is because in daily life, too, breathing through the nose is best. In addition to filtering, warming, and moisturizing the air we breathe, it gives our lungs more time to extract oxygen. As an added bonus, regularly breathing through the nose rather than the mouth is a way to counteract unwelcome habits like snoring.

INHALATION

In most systems of yoga, a correct and complete method of breathing is one where in the phase of inhalation the breath is experienced as starting from below, in the abdomen. From there it moves upward toward the top of the chest.

As mentioned earlier, complete breathing is generally considered to consist of three basic phases: the first is usually called the abdominal phase, the second the intercostal phase, and the third the chest phase.

The individual phases or types of respiration are known by other names as well. Yoga expert H. David Coulter, for example, makes a distinction between what he calls abdominal or abdomino-diaphragmatic breathing, diaphragmatic or thoraco-diaphragmatic breathing, and thoracic breathing.

In addition to being different names, they also imply different dynamics, characteristics, and functions, related to the interdependent actions of the diaphragm, lungs, rib cage, and position.

Be that as it may, none of these designations corresponds to what is actually happening from the perspective of physiology. Rather, the various terms describe our subjective experience of the breathing process.

For example, when we say abdominal breathing, it is not that we actually breathe into the abdomen. This is what we experience, an expansion of the abdomen while inhaling. But the air is in fact expanding in the lungs only.

These three phases are described separately simply for the sake of understanding, and to help us learn how to establish the correct mechanics of relaxed, complete, and effective respiration. In essence they are completely interconnected. They have to be one, integrated, continuous, spontaneous flow.

As already indicated, the first and most important phase of complete breathing is the lower region of the abdomen.

In this book, to make it simple, I am using mostly "abdominal" to indicate what I call the "below-first" phase of the inhalation.

In the beginning, or until we have learned otherwise, many of us tend to bloat the abdomen, to push it forward too much – to force its expansion. This action will immediately limit the possibility of correct, harmonious inhalation.

A simple and effective way to clearly experience the abdominal phase is to lie down on the floor, on the back, with the feet a little apart, and breathe easily. The sensation of the breath expanding into the abdomen should be quite apparent.

In this position you can feel the diaphragm lowering during inhalation and causing an abdominal expansion. During exhalation the diaphragm moves upward again, causing the abdomen to deflate.

Unfortunately, many people actually breathe exactly in a reverse way, flattening the belly when inhaling and expanding it when exhaling. This is not a healthy pattern of respiration.

Moreover, when not properly trained, or without experience and the understanding of how to do it, on inhaling and trying to expand from below first, the tendency will be to jump from abdomen to the chest and the back, in a scattered, uneven pattern.

Instead, the expansion of the lower abdomen needs to be controlled, to avoid bloating or overinflating, while the upper abdomen is allowed to also expand to the sides, without tension or forced effort. If necessary, you may find that focusing your attention on the area of the lower pubis helps you avoid the tendency to overinflate.

With practice, you can develop this skill without needing to exert active control on the lower abdomen. The correct mechanics of breathing become more spontaneous; you can relinquish control and be able to enjoy the natural flow of healthy breathing.

We can rediscover the inhalation as an upward movement of breath that can expand harmoniously.

In this diagram illustrating the kind of abdominal breathing we consider most effective for a harmonious flow of the inhalation, we can see that the movement of the expansion of the breath is shaped like an arrowhead:

The blue line formed by small blue arrows indicates the central core or shaft of the larger arrowhead shape. The small brown arrows moving diagonally upward from its sides and show the direction of the expansion of the inhalation, starting from the bottom and expanding upward and to the sides.

Inhalation progresses upward along the central shaft, and simultaneously upward and outward along the sides.

In other words, rather than merely expanding upward in the center, the movement of the inhalation also opens laterally to the sides, much like the shape of an arrowhead.

One of the easiest ways to experience a bottom-up dynamic of the inhalation, to help it start from below, is to focus your mind on the abdomen.

You can also place one or both hands there to guide your focus. Keep your presence there. The inhalation will more easily start where your presence is.

From below, the abdominal phase of breathing, the air ideally expands smoothly upward, unhindered. The rib cage expands and allows space to be created for the air to then fill the lungs: first at the level of the lower rib cage (the intercostal breathing phase), then up into the chest and upper chest.

An expansion of the back of the torso can also be experienced, because the quality of complete breathing is meant to be clearly perceived as tridimensional, expanding like an inflating balloon.

EXHALATION

Let us now look at what may be the best pattern of exhalation to support a harmonious inhalation. In reality we can train our body to breathe in different ways, and this is good, because it is also important to have flexibility in the way we breathe.

The key is to experience and try to discover without preconception what works for you, what makes your breathing flow naturally, and experience the sensation of well-being that comes with truly natural, healthy breathing.

This well-being will manifest not just as the feeling that you are breathing better, but also that your body is moving better, with less tension and with more vigor. And, most importantly, we notice that the mind is clearer, more focused yet relaxed. This condition of clarity is something very precious. It is a goal not just for people interested in yoga, but a condition that everyone deserves to be able to experience.

In Yantra Yoga, the ancient Tibetan practice with profound knowledge of the functions of breathing, exhalations start in the upper chest and move downward to the abdomen. From the top to the bottom, the breath is meant to have the same, unfragmented, fluid flow. So here, too, we will learn how to exhale smoothly and fully to infuse our respiration with a complete, harmonious flow.

This diagram illustrates the progression of an exhalation in complete breathing: first, we exhale from the chest, then from the rib cage, and then from the abdomen. The exhalation needs to be a continuous flow, without interruptions, without fragmentation. This is very important.

Inhaling from the bottom up, exhaling from the top down, in a continuous flow, we create the natural waves of Harmonious Breathing.

This diagram illustrates the pattern of exhalation from top to bottom in more detail. Here, the direction of the brown and blue arrows shows the progression of the exhalation – beginning with releasing the breath from the chest, then from the center and the sides, and finally from the abdomen. We let the air out from the center and from the sides, again describing a triangular movement.

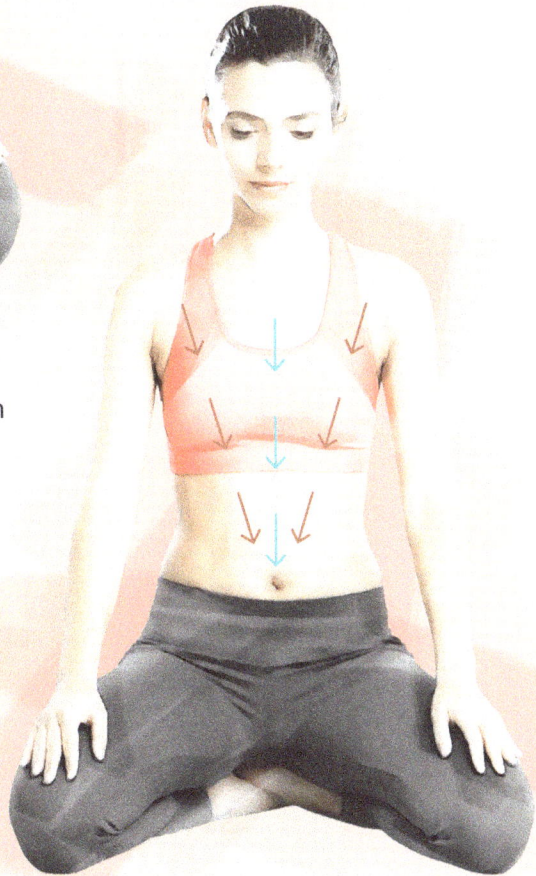

The arrowhead shape is the same as for inhalation, but both in direction and progression, the process is exactly the opposite.

Inhalation moves into exhalation and back into inhalation continuously, without being blocked or fragmented.

PAUSES

At this point, we need to acknowledge another factor that is fundamental to truly tension-free, flowing respiration: pauses. We already addressed this topic briefly in the introduction, but in this context it is worth taking a closer look at it.

In our natural breathing pattern, we have two pauses: one after inhalation and one after exhalation. We inhale and pause; we exhale and pause. We may not be aware of it, but we do.

The pattern of our respiration is correctly shaped by nature: it is like an ellipse with the two extremities corresponding to the two pauses.

Rather than being conditioned by this natural impulse to pause, which because of tension often leads to fragmented respiration, we need to take control, be aware of it, and learn how to use it, learn how to relax into it to achieve the flow of harmonious breathing.

Pauses can also be described as holds. The art and science of holding our breath is a big part of the practice of yoga, but is not the theme of this book.

"By retaining one's in-drawn breath, [energy] is fully absorbed and distributed to the entire system through the circulation of blood. [...] By pausing after the out-breath according to one's capacity, all stresses are purged and drained away. The mind remains silent and tranquil."

BKS Iyengar, Light on Life

When applied in a correct, conscious way, when we are present and aware of it, these pauses are a precious tool for helping to rid us of the tendency to block and fragment our respiration. Fragmented and tense breathing is the basis of an unbalanced condition of our energy and weakness of our elements.

Together with a smooth flow of the breath, it is equally important to have flexibility in our breathing. We can learn how to expand it and how to contract it. We do not have to be limited to short, tense breathing.

It is for this reason that we need to train our capacity, train how to expand the breathing and how to limit it, how to let it be passive and how to take active control of it.

Our goal it is not to have a "bigger" capacity of breathing just for the sake of it, but rather to develop a breathing pattern that will allow us to breathe in a healthier way, to breathe with quality.

The objective is to experience a free flowing of our breath, as much as possible unconditioned by our stress-related tensions. These tensions are stored in our body, unbalancing our energy and clouding our mind.

THE ROLE OF COMPLETE BREATHING IN YOGA

For readers who are yoga practitioners, I would like to stress the importance of coordinating complete breathing with fluid movements and consciously breathing during static postures.

Alignment is a fundamental aspect of any yoga practice, and recently many yoga teachers are expanding the concept of alignment from a purely anatomical, mechanical focus to embrace a more integral approach.

Breathing is a central factor in arriving at this more organic dimension of alignment. By working with the breath, representing the level of energy, we can arrive at the perfect alignment of body, energy, and mind.

PART 2 |

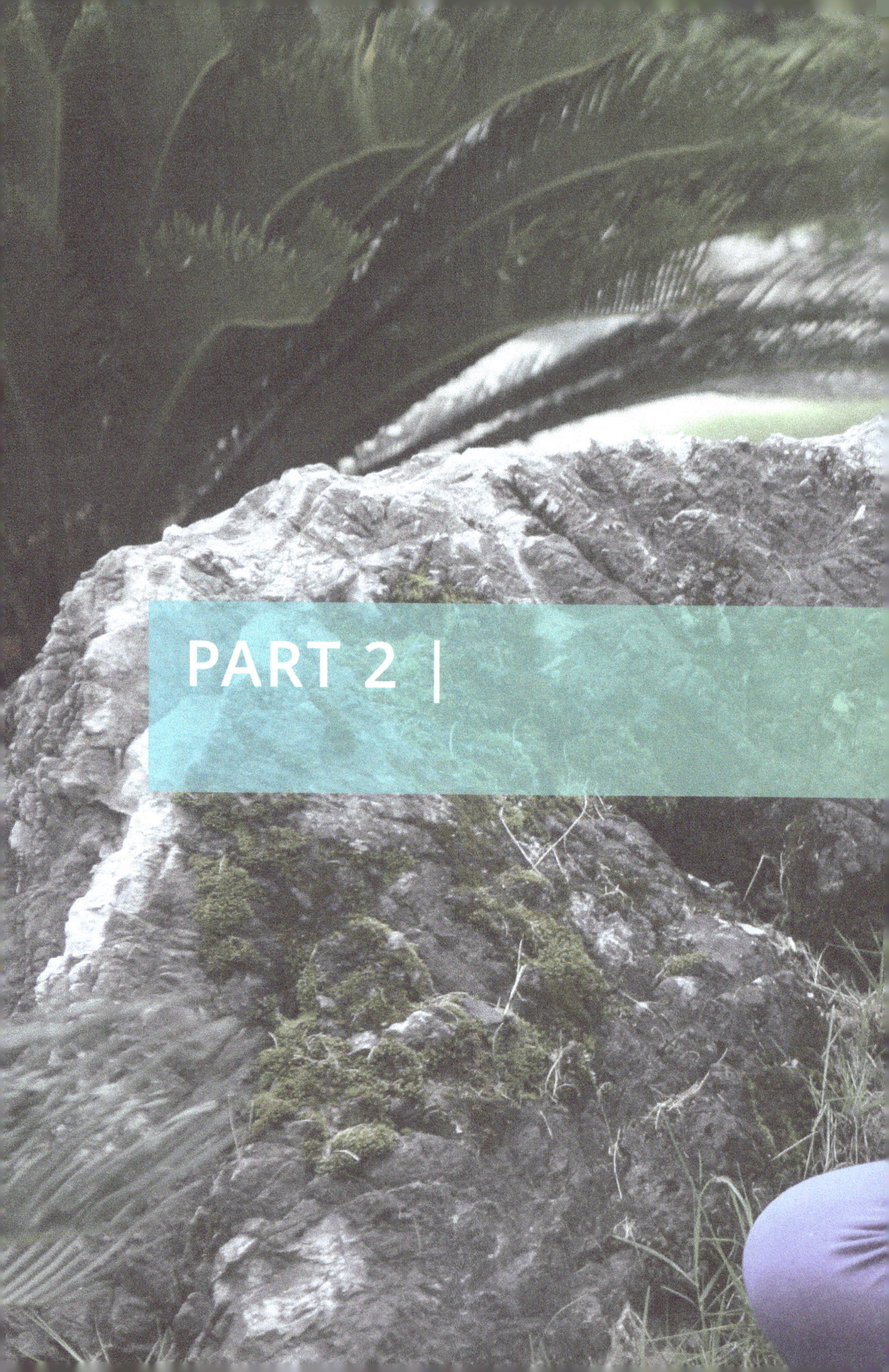

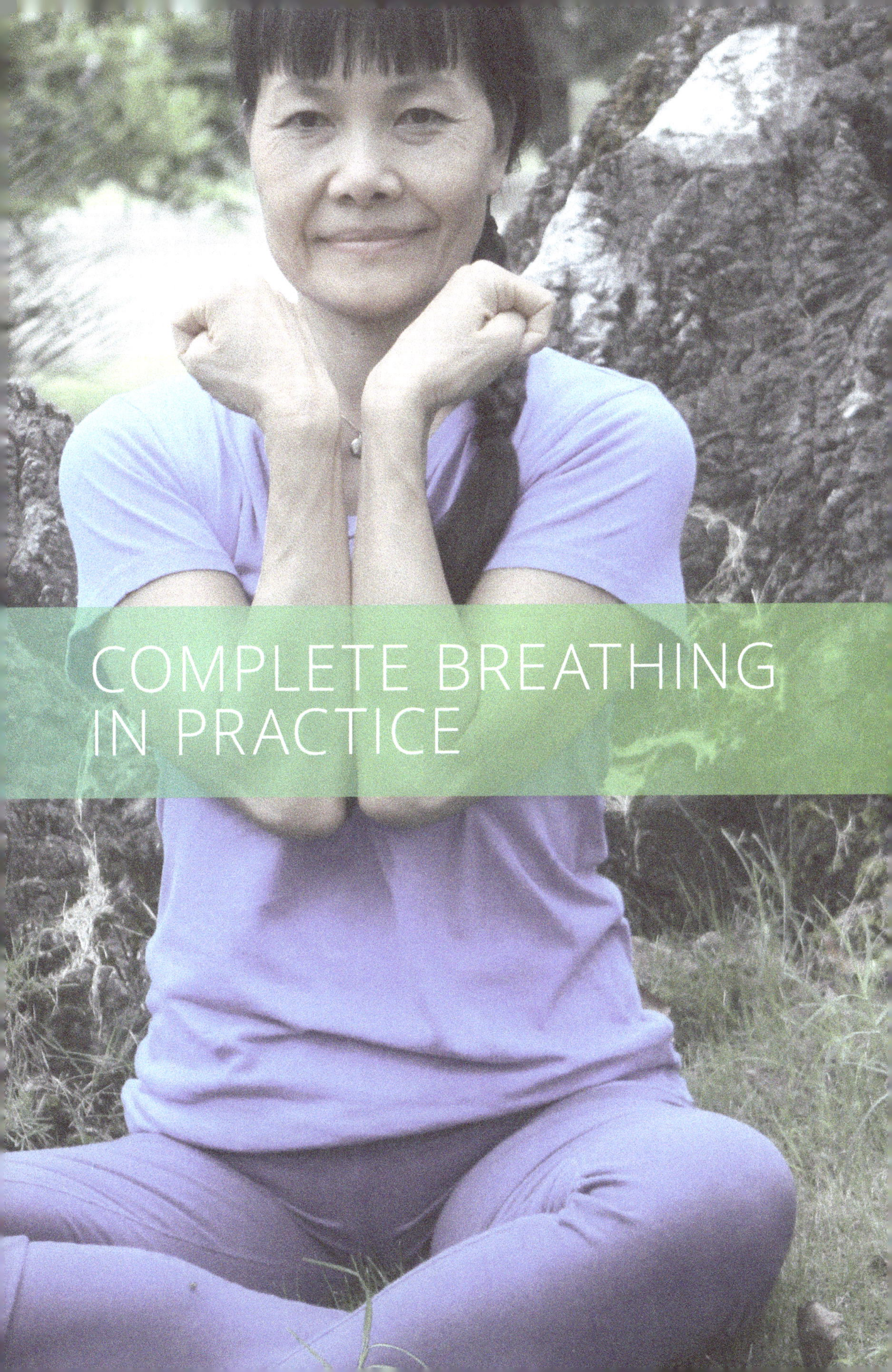

COMPLETE BREATHING
IN PRACTICE

HARMONIOUS BREATHING

Relaxed, complete breathing is characterized by inhalations that expand upward easily, naturally, without forcing or bloating. The exhalations are unhindered, smooth, and long. Complete breathing promotes health and well-being. It is the key to a positive, relaxed state of mind, sound sleep, good digestion, stabilized blood pressure, and countless other health benefits.

The Harmonious Breathing method uses an experiential approach, taking you through the individual stages of complete breathing to teach you how to breathe in a complete, fluid way. In effect, by doing these exercises you are teaching your body how to breathe well.

Some Harmonious Breathing exercises are

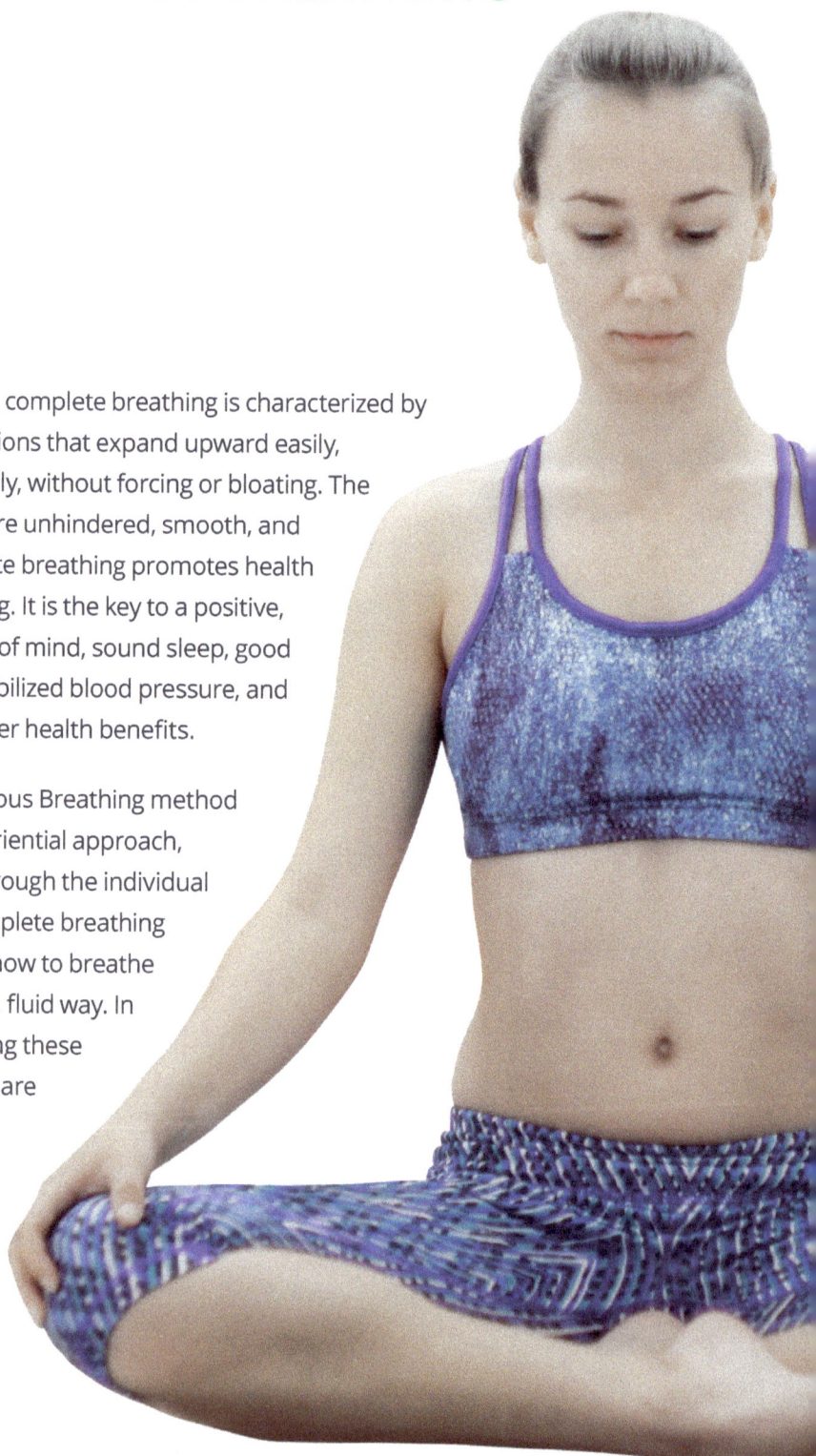

quite simple. Some are more engaging, and some a bit challenging. Some are passive, static, and some are more dynamic, more energetic. The variety creates the foundation for experiencing a synergistic interaction of different qualities of breathing. Everyone can find something useful here, something suited to his or her character and capacities.

You can practice on any firm, level surface or chair. For comfort, you can use some padding, but not too thick. An excessively soft, uneven surface could be harmful for the spine.

A number of these exercises will be easier for people who have a little experience in yoga or other breathwork or bodywork, but the basic ones – indicated with the icon for "easy" – are absolutely for everyone: anyone can train and develop a more harmonious way of breathing and have a concrete, real benefit in daily life.

Although at first sight some of the sequences may appear quite similar to others, such as various versions of the Bridge and the Cat, slight variations in some aspects of the exercise and the modality and timing of the breathing emphasize entirely different phases of the breathing.

Other groups of exercises give you a chance to explore and expand the experience of the four phases, teaching you how to coordinate them more effectively and just relax with the breath. The Four Keys is a set of exceptionally simple and yet powerful exercises that can be used on their own as the basis of a quick tune-up session or combined with others to unlock whichever phase you happen to be working on.

As explained in appendix 2, once you are a little familiar with the material in this book, you will easily be able to put together a routine to suit your time, flexibility, and preferences. You can start by choosing one of the suggested routines and then gradually add and subtract exercises to personalize your session. Essentially, anything more than a condensed, quick routine should include some warm-ups before moving to the core exercises. A large selection of warm-ups is provided in appendix 1.

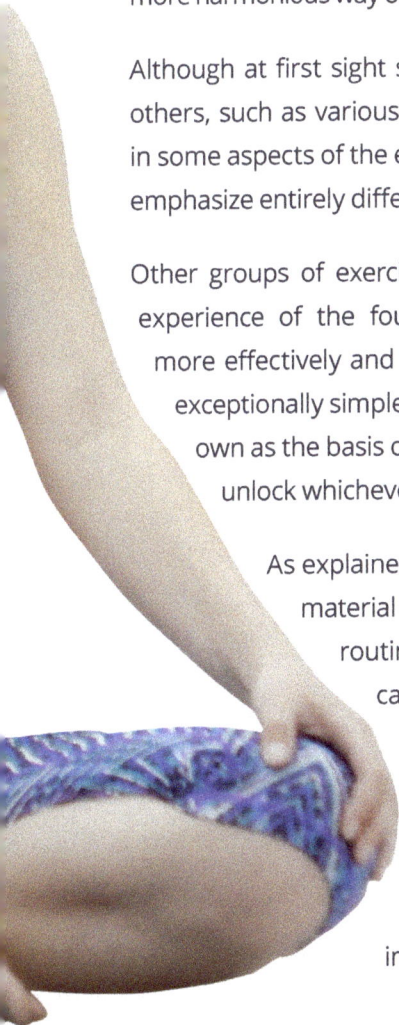

KEY TO EXERCISES BY LEVEL

To help you choose the exercises that are right for you, each of the core Harmonious Breathing exercises and warm-ups in this book is also identified by level of difficulty according to the following key:

1. 👍 EASY

These exercises are for everyone. They are so simple that even someone with physical challenges and no experience can use them to discover how to breathe better and relax the tensions in the body.

Many of the easy exercises have a passive quality, where there is not really anything to do except breathe.

2. 👌 MODERATE

These exercises are generally a bit more dynamic and demanding but are still gentle.

3. ☝ CHALLENGING

The challenging exercises are a bit more stimulating; even experienced yoga practitioners will find them pleasantly engaging.

POSITIONS USED IN HARMONIOUS BREATHING

When we work with our breathing, the correct position while sitting or standing is very important.

This is especially true for seated practice. It is always crucial that your spine is straight and aligned and that you feel comfortable. In fact, any comfortable position with the back straight is good for practicing breathing, whether you are sitting on the floor or on a chair.

As with any bodywork, it is worth mentioning that most of the exercises described here are best done on an empty stomach, or at least two or three hours after a meal.

"Establishing an upright relationship to gravity, in the deepest sense, is less about exerting the correct muscular effort than it is about discovering and releasing the habitual muscular effort that is obstructing the natural tendency of the body to be supported all on its own."

Leslie Kaminoff, Yoga Anatomy

It is important to be relaxed but alert and present, aware.

Several positions are possible, from the most challenging, like the lotus position, to simpler ones.

When necessary you can use various kinds of supports to help sustain the position correctly. If it helps to keep your spine straight, you can use a prop such as a firm pillow, a folded blanket, or a rolled towel, or sit on a chair.

In addition to keeping your spine straight, the main thing is to ensure that your sides are well controlled, that they are firm and straight, and that you do not slouch backward.

Here are some examples of the more commonly used sitting positions, without and with props:

Easy

With a prop

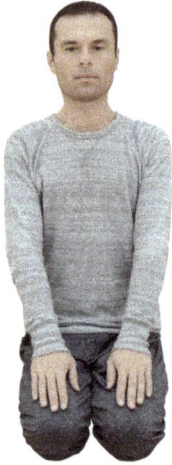

If you feel pain on the tops of your feet, you can put a blanket or a towel under them. Kneeling makes it easier to keep the back straight. Push the navel slightly forward and pull the chin in a little.

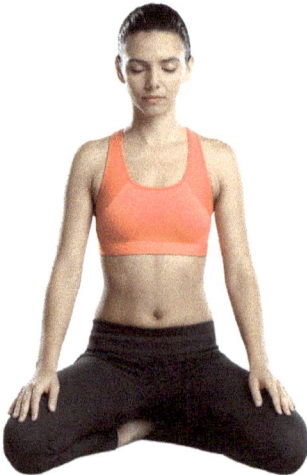

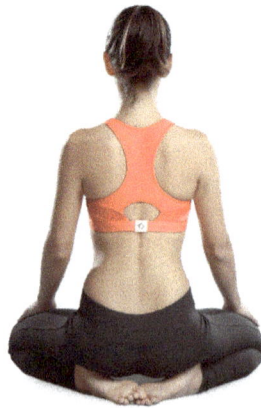

Kneeling with the knees open is an easy and good alternative. Put one foot on top of the other. When necessary to help keep your spine straight, you can use a prop such as a firm pillow, a blanket, or a towel.

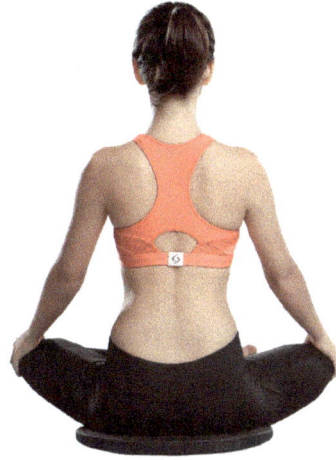

Half lotus

With a prop

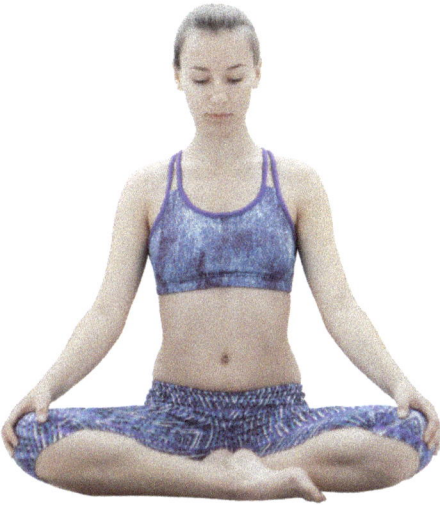

Relaxed half lotus

Lotus

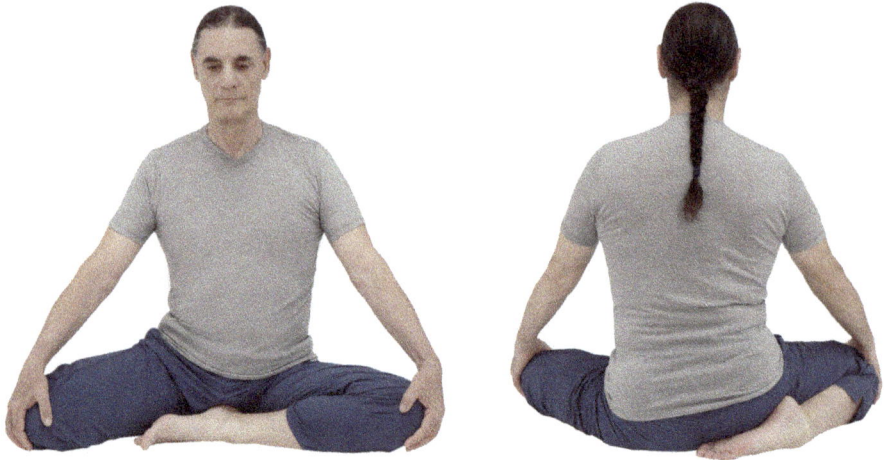

One leg bent in front

One leg bent in front, the other behind (be sure to alternate sides regularly if you choose this position).

Supports can include blankets, cushions or pillows, and yoga props.

In general, a prop that is too high and soft is not ideal. Often, a relatively thin, but firm prop is better – just enough to help tilt the pelvis forward and align the spine.

You can also practice any of the seated exercises on a chair, with or without props. For example, placing a rolled towel behind the small of your back helps ensure the correct alignment.

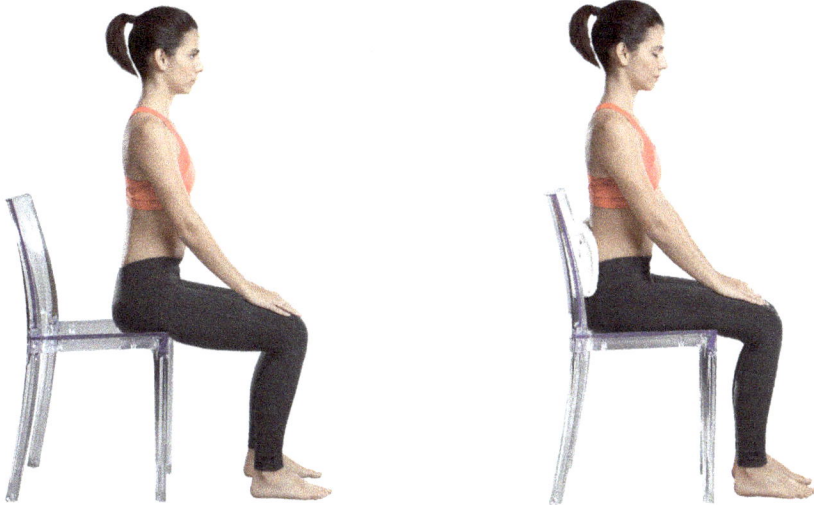

Whichever position you choose, what is most important is that you feel relaxed and at the same time present, with your position firm and steady.

We will also be using various reclining positions to train the breathing and make it more flexible:

To ensure a correct alignment, the knees should be open and feet pointed outward, arms along the sides or hands on the abdomen and the chest.

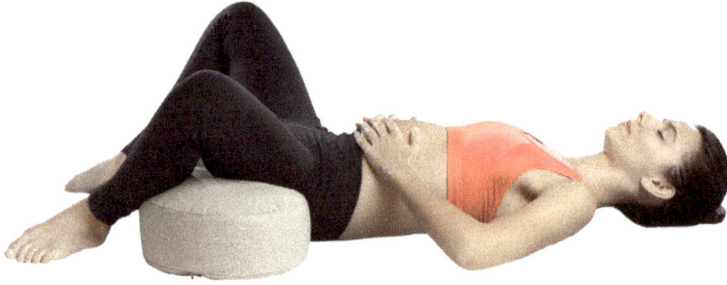

The position will be even more comfortable if you place a pillow under each knee.

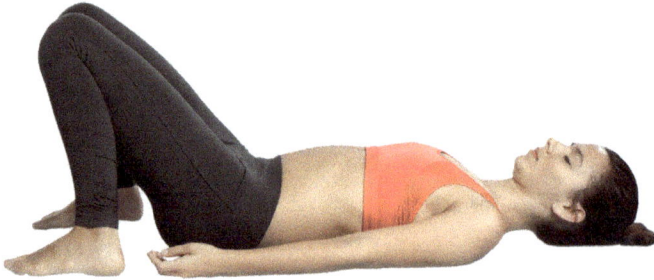

If keeping the knees open gets tiring, you can bring them together and point the feet inward.

For complete relaxation, for instance at the end of a session, simply lie on your back with your legs and arms loosely open to the sides.

THE RIGHT BEGINNING: PURIFICATION BREATHING

EXPLANATION AND POINTERS

Anytime we inhale or exhale in a tense and uneven way, certain subtle impurities accumulate in our body. We are especially prone to adopt this type of breathing when we are distracted, stressed, or conditioned by emotions, in particular negative ones.

Over time, we then develop a pattern of contracted, fragmented breathing, and when this happens, the breath loses its natural harmony and we create a condition of imbalance in our life energy force.

Purification Breathing is a method to purify and correct this negative condition of accumulated stale, impure air, and so coordinate and strengthen our energy.

In this practice it is essential to inhale well and fully, not simply relying on our normal, almost automatic way of breathing. We need to try to do more, expand more, but without creating tension. We need to be active, present, but without forcing.

As important as it is to inhale fully and harmoniously, in this exercise the main emphasis is on exhaling actively, thoroughly, and deeply – expelling as much of the stale, impure air as possible – because this is how it unfolds its beneficial effect.

If practiced in the morning, Purification Breathing will give you a cleansing and tune up of your energy to start a new day. It will leave you feeling both relaxed and energized.

THE SEVEN-POINT POSTURE

When we are working with our respiration, a proper position is fundamental for coordinating our energy and allowing a harmonious flow of the respiration. The Seven-Point Posture applied in Yantra Yoga defines the essential characteristics of the ideal seated posture:

1. Legs crossed
2. Hands on the knees
3. Tongue touching the palate
4. Eyes, lips, and teeth naturally relaxed
5. Spine straight as an arrow (tip of the nose aligned with the navel)
6. Chest and shoulders open
7. Entire body relaxed and controlled at the same time

Once again, the essence of the correct position is both to have the back straight and to be comfortable, so any position that allows for these two aspects will do. It is not a fundamental requirement to sit cross-legged on the floor. Any of the seated postures introduced above is acceptable, as long as the back is straight.

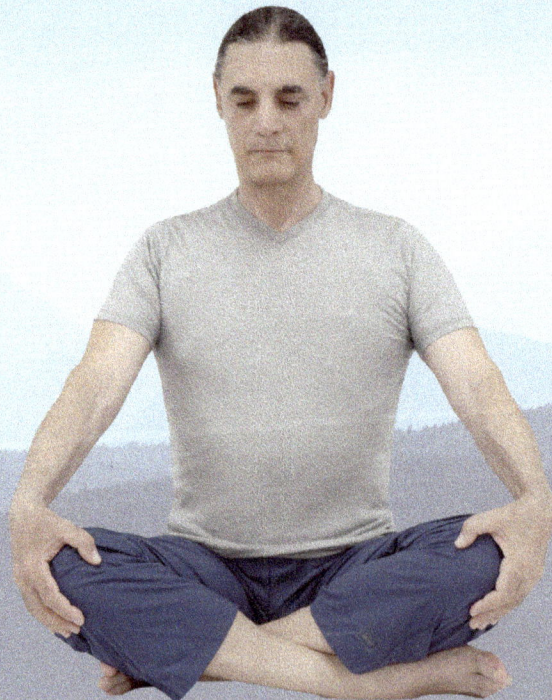

THE PRACTICE

This is a short version of a practice done in Yantra Yoga to eliminate accumulated stale air.

Seated in a comfortable position with the back properly aligned, inhale slowly, directly and completely, fully opening the chest.

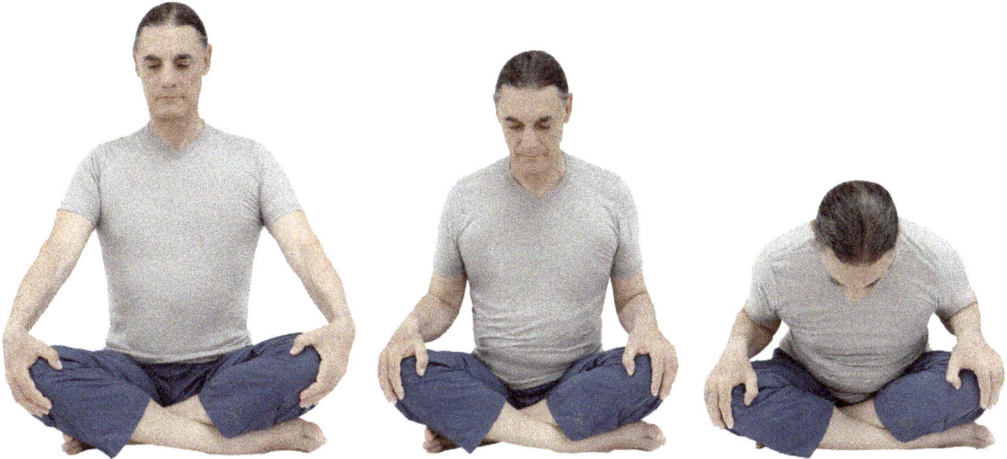

Start to exhale the upper air without changing your position. Then, keeping your back straight, continue to exhale while bending forward from the hips.

A simple sequence of movements will help you experientially understand what it means to have your back correctly aligned and "straight as an arrow":

Inhale, extending the arms straight and all the way up, parallel along the sides of the head, and opening the chest and shoulders well. Then exhale, lowering your hands back to your knees, but without dropping the shoulders, keeping the sides active.

A correct alignment of the position is fundamental. When you feel you are relaxed yet present, your body is controlled but without tension. The position will then be the perfect vehicle for the smooth, correct expansion of the breathing – and not an obstacle.

As you come forward, bring your elbows close to your sides. This will help you exhale completely and eliminate all of the stale air.

If you are able, and are in a position that will allow it, bend forward as far as you can, making sure to keep the back straight, finishing the exhalation with your forehead toward or touching the ground.

It is important to start the forward movement from the base of the spine, or more precisely from the level of the navel, not from the head or the shoulders. This will keep the movement easier and more fluid. It is also gentler on the spine.

After exhaling, while bent forward, pause a little, keeping the lungs empty, before inhaling and gradually moving back to the starting position.

If it helps, you can start to come up while still empty, just for a moment, until you feel where the inhalation can best begin in a smooth and easy way.

Repeat this sequence a total of three times.

After each exhalation, be sure to inhale well, expanding the air up to the chest, filling slowly and completely from bottom to top. Be aware of starting to inhale from below. Keep your mind there.

If in the beginning it proves difficult to breathe through the nostrils, you can either inhale through the nostrils and exhale through the mouth or directly and vigorously inhale and exhale from the mouth, making sure to concentrate on a thorough exhalation.

FREE-FLOWING BREATHING

In most Harmonious Breathing exercises, inhalations and exhalations should be long and free from control, without any blockage or constriction in the throat. In other words, on the inhalation, the air feels as if it goes directly from nostrils into the lungs. If you feel any constriction in the glottis, or note any rasping or coughing sound, release the tension so that the breath is smooth and unhindered.

When inhaling, we fill the lungs gradually from the bottom to the top, as if we were filling a vase with water.

When exhaling, we first empty the top of the lungs and last the lower part of the lungs. It is crucial to exhale correctly and fully.

The ideal shape of the inhalation and the exhalation is sometimes compared to a grain of barley, starting slowly, opening to a stronger flow, and tapering off to a smooth, gradual end.

The mind is present, relaxed but alert and focused on the unified flow of breathing and movement. This is mindful respiration.

Applying this method will help purify, coordinate, and harmonize your breathing, the function of your elements, and your vital energy.

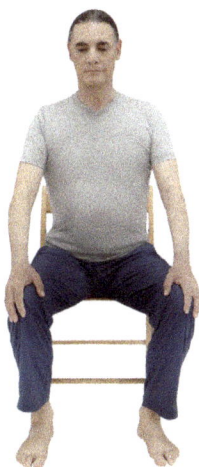

As a result, your mind can relax more easily and at the same time be alert, less distracted, and less conditioned by stressful thoughts and emotions.

The Purification Breathing exercise can also be done sitting in a chair. On the exhalations, simply bend forward as far as comfortable, with the back engaged and the elbows moving close to the sides.

DEVELOPING THE ABDOMINAL PHASE

n the abdominal phase of complete breathing, the lower part of the lungs fills up first while the diaphragm is swinging downward. This is very important and needs to be trained well. In the beginning it is necessary to "unlock" your abdominal breathing. The following exercises help you make it work more efficiently.

Done correctly, abdominal breathing expands in the abdomen naturally. A common mistake is to push the abdomen out or bloat it: what we are striving for is a natural expansion. To achieve that, we have to try to dissolve and overcome the tensions that block the possibility of expanding properly.

Abdominal breathing plays an important role in activating the parasympathetic nervous system, triggering what is called the relaxation response. This is why abdomen-focused breathing exercises are often a central part of stress and trauma therapy. So we can understand how crucial it is to learn how to expand our abdominal breathing capacity. In addition to supporting our development of a complete breathing pattern, it can help us overcome moments of anxiety and stress.

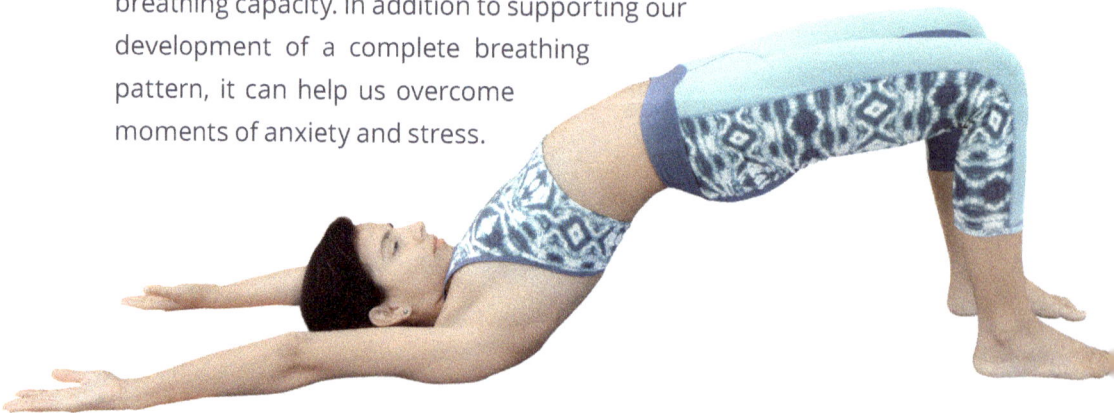

EXERCISE 1: CHIN TUCK

👍 EASY

This is a simple exercise that will give you an initial experience of "below first" breathing.

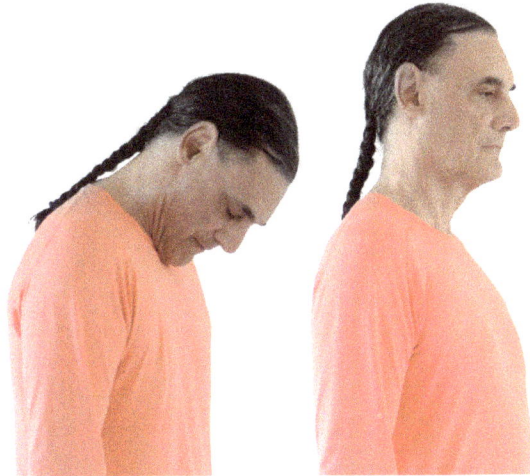

Sitting or standing with the back aligned and controlled, exhale, bringing the chin toward the chest. Keeping the chin tucked into the chest, inhale through the nostrils, and you will automatically experience a mostly diaphragmatic inhalation.

Inhale and exhale a few times this way.

If toward the end of an inhalation you untuck your chin and straighten the head, the breath is free to gently rise into the chest, without, however, entering the upper chest too much. You will have a clear experience of an open expansion that is free of tension at the base of the throat.

The position of the tucked chin restricts the flow of breath into the upper chest. This ensures that during the process of inhalation the breath expands mostly in the abdomen.

But sometimes we need something more physically engaging to unlock the abdominal breathing.

We need an exercise that will make breathing into the abdomen almost completely automatic; something that will just make it happen, even if it means overexpanding a little.

The Bridge – in its various versions – is a highly effective tool for developing the abdominal phase. Before doing any of the Bridge exercises in this section, you might find it helpful to practice the related Bridge warm-ups (see appendix 1).

EXERCISE 2: THE SHAPING BRIDGE

👍 MODERATE

The Shaping Bridge gives you a precise experience of an abdominally focused expansion that is already partially shaped for the correct application of complete breathing.

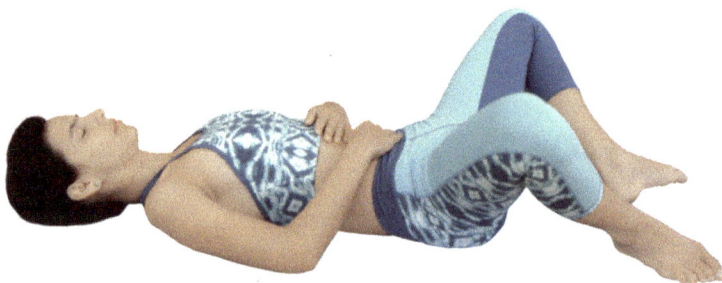

Start with relaxed breathing while lying on the ground with your knees open, heels in front of the buttocks, and feet pointing outward, allowing the outer edges of the feet to rest on the ground. Focus your attention on the abdominal breathing.

In this position, because of the particular dynamics involved in the movements of the diaphragm, it is possible to have a clearer experience of unhindered abdominal (diaphragmatic) breathing.

You can gently place both your hands on your abdomen to help focus your presence and awareness. Rest like this for a few rounds of breath.

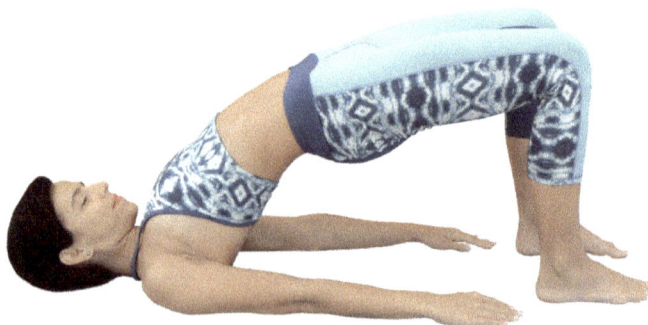

Now bring your heels closer to your buttocks, leaving your arms along the sides, and then arch your spine upward as gradually as possible, continuing to inhale and exhale, but without unduly forcing.

At this point you are ready for the central part of the exercise, with three different alternatives to choose from:

1. Hold onto your ankles and stay arched.

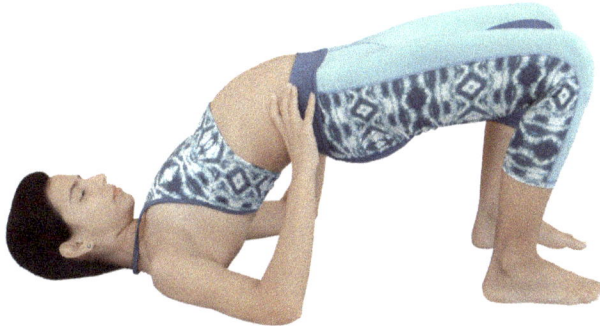

2. Stay arched, supporting your weight on your elbows, with your hands on the waist, thumbs on the hips, and fingers on the sides.

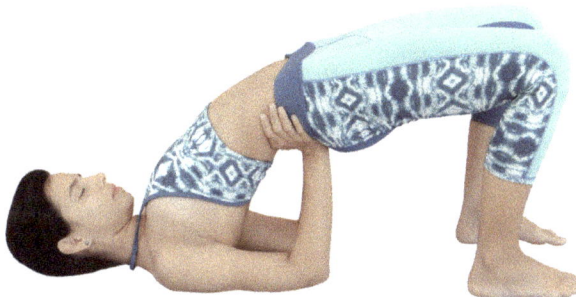

3. Support the arched position with the weight on your elbows and the palms of your hands.

In this last version, you will have to bring your elbows closer together, and you will also gain more height. This is the best "shaped" of the three alternatives, but also the most difficult.

When in the position, no matter which of the three you choose, breathe slowly and deeply through the nostrils, without forcing, expanding the abdomen, breathing fluidly and fully, taking your time as you inhale and exhale for a maximum of three to five rounds of breathing.

GETTING THE FULL BENEFITS OF THE BRIDGE

In this and the other Bridge exercises, including the ones in the warm-ups, when circumstances permit, try to stay in the central position with your pelvis raised for as long one or two minutes, continuing the same relaxed and calm breathing pattern. The prolonged, but gentle stretch is highly beneficial for the quads (the muscle group on the front of the thigh) and the psoas (the all-important yet often neglected muscle that connects the upper and lower body). One minute is generally sufficient, but if you manage to hold the position for two minutes you activate the fascia, making it even more effective. This principle is valid for all types of gentle stretches.

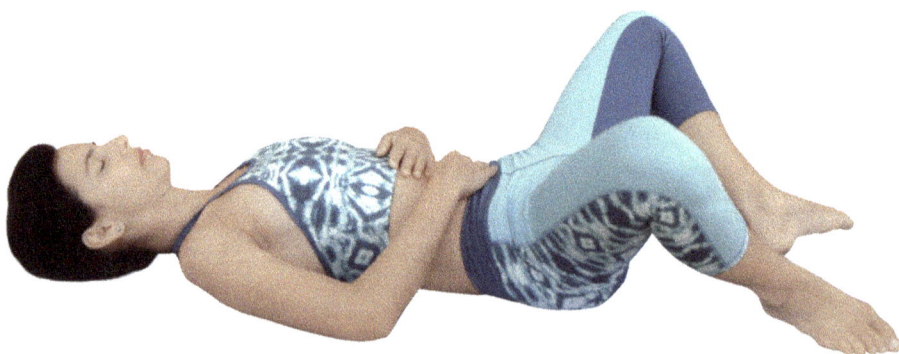

Then exhale as you lower your back to the ground, resuming the previous position with your knees wide open and hands on the abdomen. If you feel any strain in this position you can bring the knees together, leaving the feet wider than the knees.

Continue with a spontaneous and relaxed breathing rhythm, closely observing the movement of the abdominal breathing. Stay here for a few breaths, relaxing and observing.

Then rise back up into the arched position and breathe fully and fluidly.

Return to the position on the ground and observe how the exercise you just did influences the way the abdominal breathing is now expanding. Relax into it, letting it be as spontaneous as possible.

This exercise is particularly useful because it creates the ideal conditions for you to breathe abdominally, diaphragmatically. It helps you become aware of how this fundamental phase of complete breathing actually feels, enabling you to then apply it in other situations as well.

When you breathe in this way you might still distend the abdomen a little too much (especially the lower abdomen) instead of controlling the expansion.

Don't worry – we're still in the training phase. The next few exercises will shape the lower breathing more correctly.

During complete breathing the expansion should be easy and natural, without forcing or bloating, opening mostly into the upper abdomen.

Notice how this exercise opens your awareness of abdominal, diaphragmatic breathing.

After a few rounds of breath, with both hands placed on the abdomen and focusing only on the abdominal breathing, move one hand to the chest and feel the air expanding under both hands, starting from below and expanding upward.

After practicing in this way you can introduce a pause, after the exhalation, just for a moment, before smoothly moving into the next inhalation. You can do this a few times. Each time be sure to transition smoothly from the pause into the inhalation phase.

Finally, come back to letting the inhalation phase of the breath expand mostly in the abdomen, without controlling it in any way, and relax into it.

EXERCISE 3: THE OPEN BRIDGE

👍 MODERATE

This exercise is similar to the previous one, but focuses more specifically on exhaling from the top down and inhaling from the bottom up.

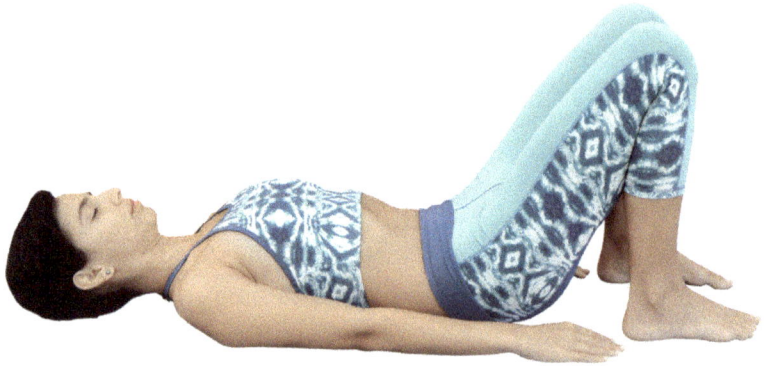

Start by lying on your back with your arms along the sides and heels near your buttocks.

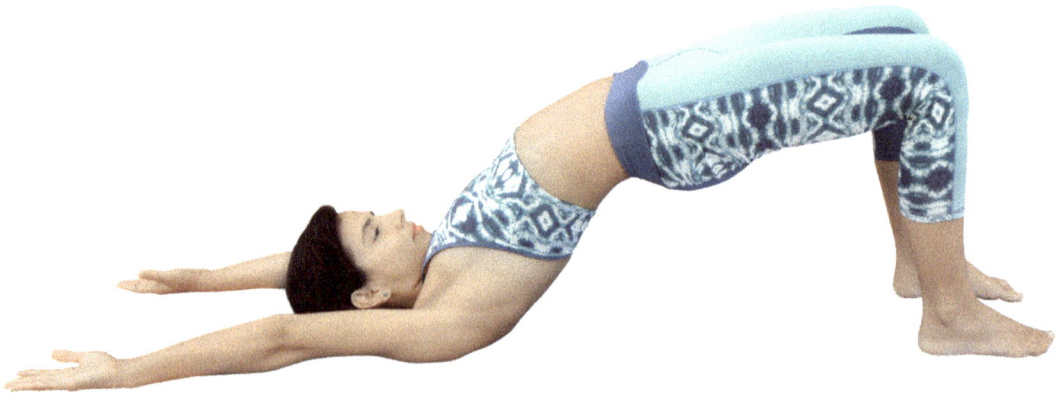

Unlike in the Shaping Bridge, this time, as you inhale and lift your hips up to arch your back, stretch your arms straight up and over your head to the floor.

The arc described by the arms, the arching of the back, and the flow of the breath should all happen simultaneously and be harmoniously synchronized.

Now, keeping your torso well arched, start to exhale as you first bring your hands together over the head and then raise your extended arms directly above your eyes. This movement makes it easier to start exhaling the upper chest air first.

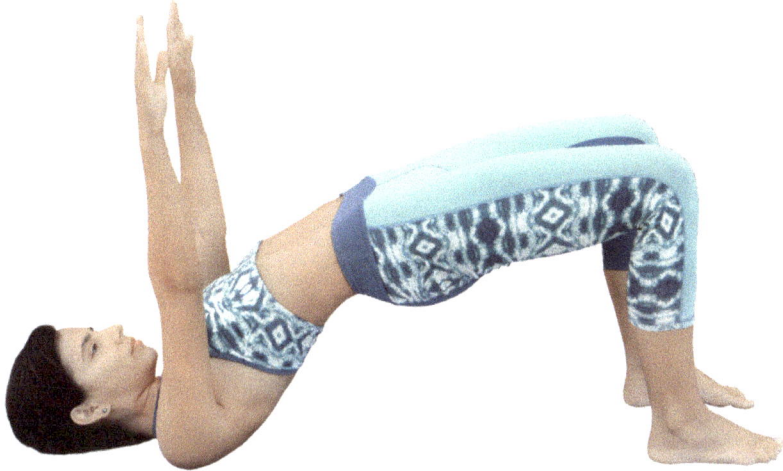

Holding this same position, inhale, noticing the mostly abdominal inhalation. Then exhale, gradually lowering the arms along the sides and the back to the floor.

Repeat this exercise a few times, observing its effects on exhaling from the chest and inhaling from the abdomen.

The Open Bridge is a highly useful tool for starting to train the "chest-exhalation-first" approach since the forward movement of the arms together with the action of gravity makes it almost automatic.

It also produces a clear experience of a well-coordinated abdominal inhalation.

EXERCISE 4: SUPPORTED BRIDGE

👍 MODERATE

This exercise, done with the aid of props, is easy to do and extremely useful for relaxing and relieving even difficult problems of the spine.

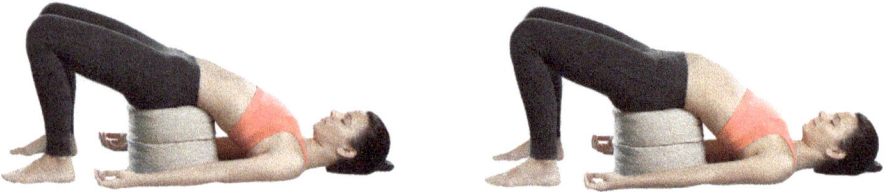

Lie on your back with your heels near your buttocks and place one or more pillows or blankets under your buttocks to support your spine. The props should be firm and placed in such a manner that you feel no strain and the arch is comfortable.

Alternatively, you can lie on the floor and rest your feet and lower legs on a chair or on a bed. This last variation of the position, besides being particularly helpful for experiencing, training, and practicing abdominal breathing, is also very good for your back.

As in the Shaping Bridge, once you are comfortable in the position, breathe slowly and deeply, but without forcing, through the nostrils, expanding the abdomen, breathing fully, but without forcing and taking your time – inhaling and exhaling for three to five rounds of breathing. You can also stay longer, especially if you want to relax and pamper your back.

When you finish any of these reclining exercises, come out of the position carefully; you can roll to one side and use your hands to support you as you come up to sitting.

EXERCISE 5: CONTRACTING AND RELEASING

CHALLENGING

This is a particularly effective method for unlocking your abdominal breathing. The position, the movement, and the precise mechanics of the exercise allow us to induce an "automatic" abdominal expansion during inhalation.

No matter how briefly you do it, it is advisable to perform this exercise only on an empty stomach, and only if you feel very comfortable about it. This kind of strong abdominal contraction is best avoided if you have any kind of hernia or a chronic gastrointestinal problem such as an ulcer.

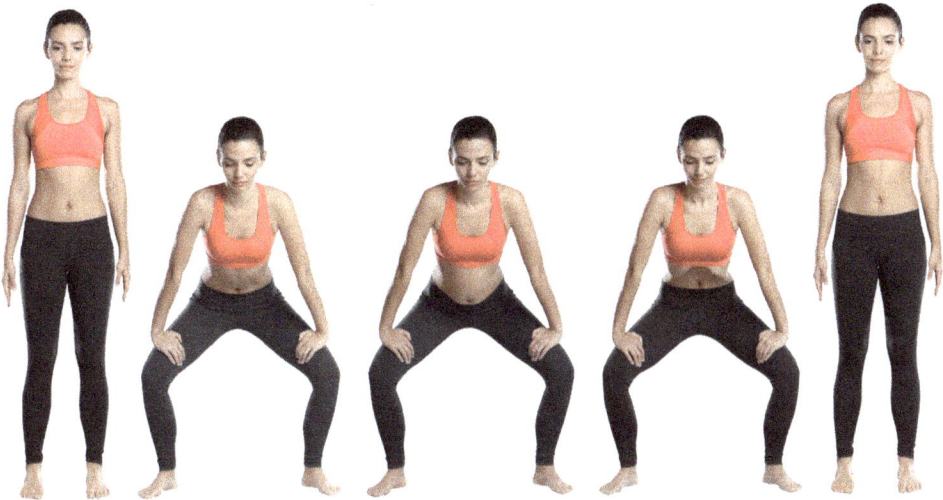

Stand with the legs well apart, hands on the thighs above the knees. The back is straight and the chin slightly toward the chest.

Exhale completely, actively bringing the navel toward the spine by contracting the abdominal muscles. Then immediately release the contraction of the abdominal muscles and let the abdomen expand with the impulse of the inhalation.

Repeat no more than three times.

Then, remaining in the posture, after the exhalation, instead of immediately inhaling, firmly pull the navel toward the spine. When contracting the navel, be sure to just pull it straight toward the spine, without also pulling it upward.

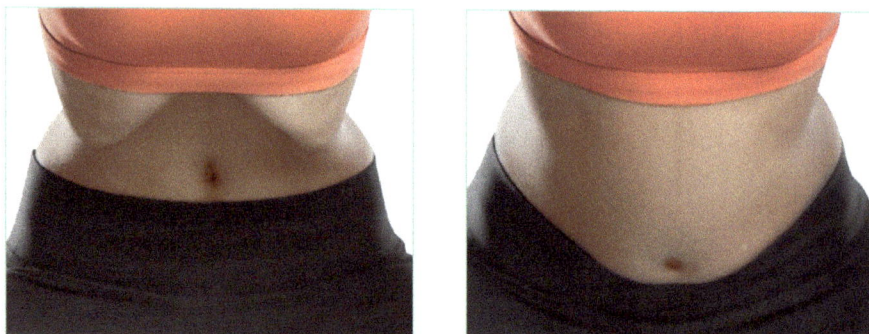

Then let go of the backward contraction and allow the abdomen to expand as you start to inhale.

You can end the inhalation by coming into an upright standing position with your arms along the sides. Breathe normally a few times if you need to.

Exhale deeply as you bend forward to begin this phase of the exercise again, repeating no more than three times.

Finally, repeat as before, again no more than three times, but in this phase, after strongly contracting the abdomen, pause and hold empty. Stay empty for a count of two, three, or four seconds while still contracting, then let go – and experience the sensation of the air rushing into the abdomen and expanding it.

It should be noted that what we are describing here is not what is actually happening from the point of view of the anatomy and physiology of breathing, but rather reflects the subjective experience.

In each phase of this exercise it is important that at the moment of inhalation you do not focus on taking the air in. Instead, just release the abdomen and let the air rush in to fill the void.

When we are performing abdominal, or diaphragmatic, breathing, the descent of the diaphragm during inhalation is emphasized, creating a more efficient vacuum in the thorax that "pulls" more air into the lungs. In contrast, during exhalation the dome of the diaphragm moves upward more actively than in shallow breathing.

In addition to not performing this kind of exercise after a meal, it is important not to repeat it too many times in one session. If we overdo it, the freshness of the experience will be overshadowed by the onset of fatigue.

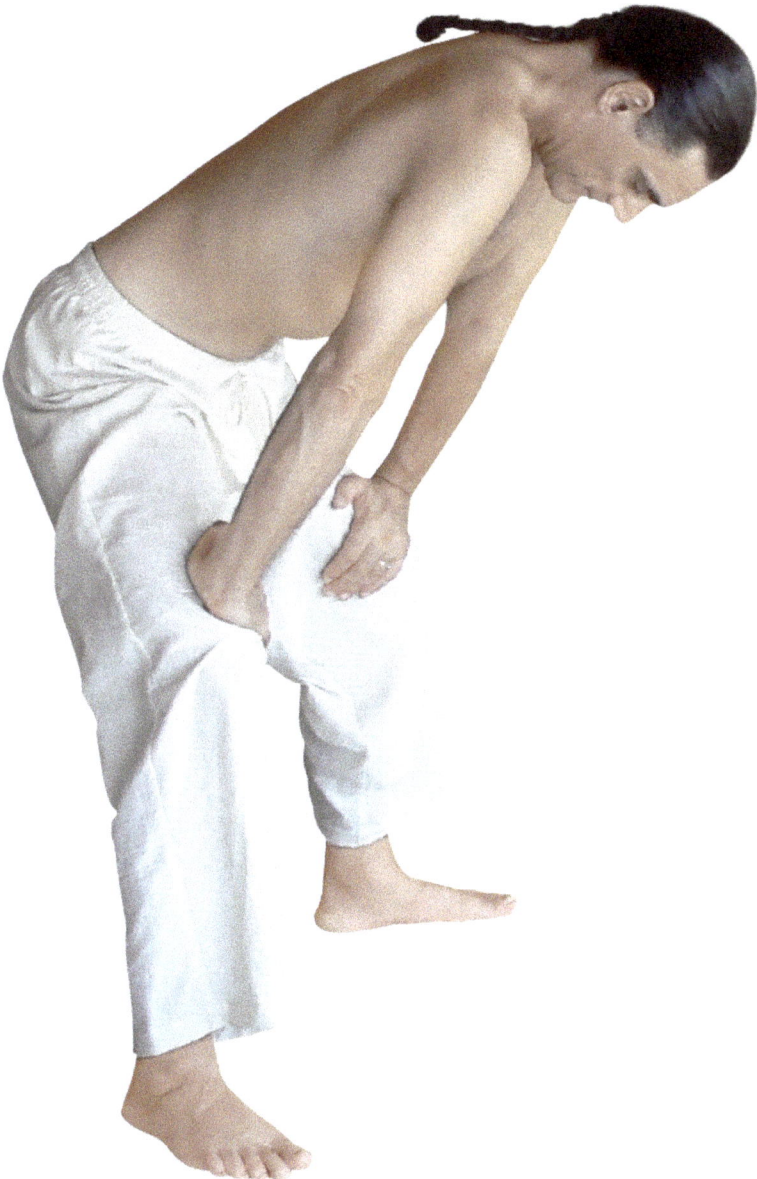

EXERCISE 6: THE ABDOMINAL CAT

👍 MODERATE

The Cat is another exercise that can help you unlock, train, and develop abdominal breathing. The Cat is also included in the warm-ups section of this book, but here we incorporate phases of empty hold so we can experience the dynamics of abdominal expansion when we inhale and release the contraction.

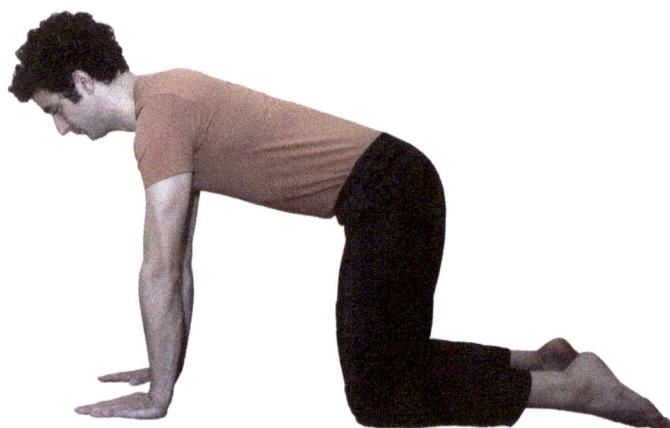

Begin by coming to all fours, with your knees and hands shoulder width apart and arms straight.

First inhale and exhale smoothly a few times.

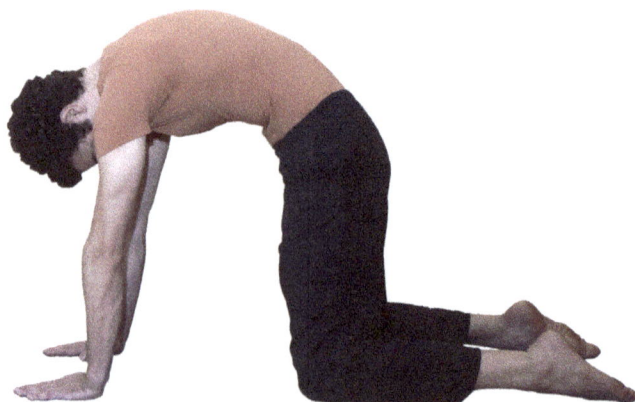

Then exhale, bringing your head between your stretched arms and arching the back like a cat.

Inhale again, lowering the navel toward the ground and raising the head up. Continue toward a full inhalation while rolling the head further back.

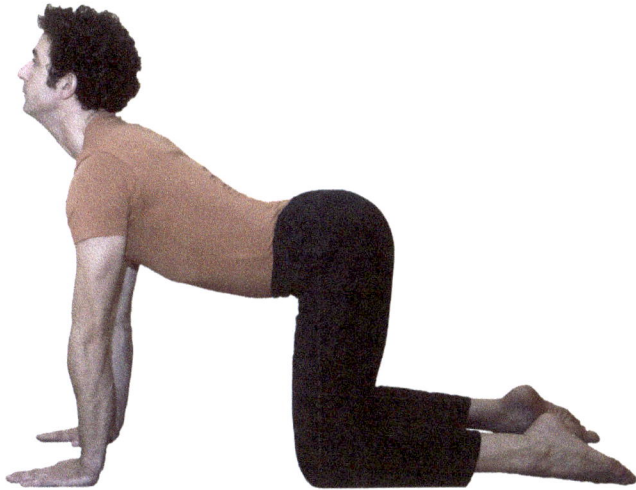

Now exhale well, again arching your back like a cat, but instead of inhaling again immediately, pause, staying empty of breath as you draw the navel toward the spine and focusing mainly on the abdomen below the navel.

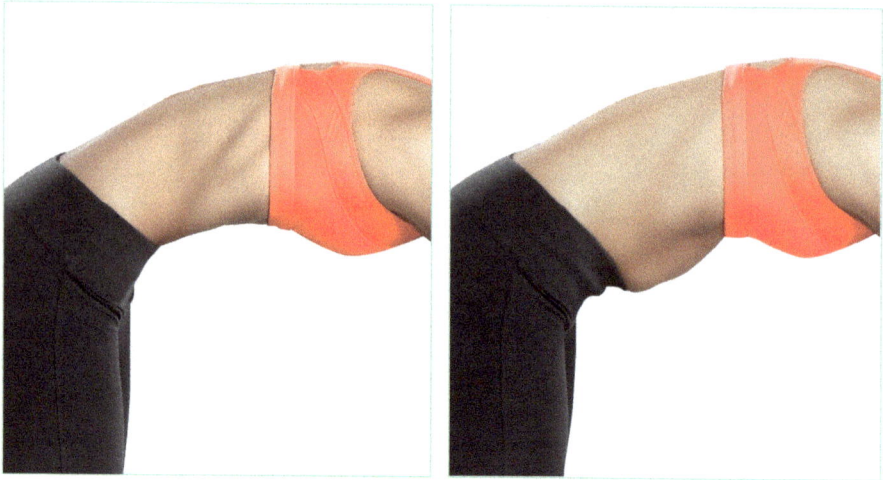

Hold empty for two, three, or four counts, then – keeping the chin tucked, and without moving the spine – release the contraction of the abdomen and let the air flood into the diaphragm, experiencing an automatic abdominal expansion.

Once you get a feel for this automatic abdominal-first expansion and understand the mechanism, you can complete the full inhalation by arching the back and raising the head a little more, continuing to inhale and arch back after the abdominal expansion is complete.

Then inhale and exhale normally before you repeat the sequence for a maximum of three to five times.

DEVELOPING THE INTERCOSTAL PHASE

The following exercises will teach you how to free the flow of the breath and guide it upward. To do this we "shape" the breath, embedding the right characteristics and mechanics of the breathing into each aspect of the entire process of respiration.

The intercostal phase of complete breathing allows the breath to expand in the middle part of the lungs and in so doing expand mostly in the mid-lower part of the rib cage. The expansion of the inhalation into the lower ribs relaxes tensions in the diaphragm and aids in the upward movement of air into the chest.

In learning these exercises, keep in mind the example of the arrowhead shape made up of smaller central and lateral arrows. As explained earlier, it represents the ideal direction of the upward expansion of the breathing, unified in a single, harmonious flow.

The upward movement follows two main directions simultaneously: along the central shaft and along the two sides of the arrowhead shape.

EXERCISE 1: BOTTOM-UP CENTRAL EXPANSION

👍 EASY

In the first exercise for the intercostal phase, we experience, train, and develop mainly the upward central movement of inhalation. The placement of the hands guides and shapes the dynamics of the abdominal breathing in such a way that even if you make the common mistake of trying to bloat in an attempt to expand the abdomen, the movement itself will correct you and help you form the right shape and dynamics.

It bears repeating that expanding the abdomen too much is not the ideal way to start a complete cycle of breathing. We should never bloat the abdomen. But we need full abdominal input in order to properly shape the breathing, and learning this is exactly the purpose of these exercises.

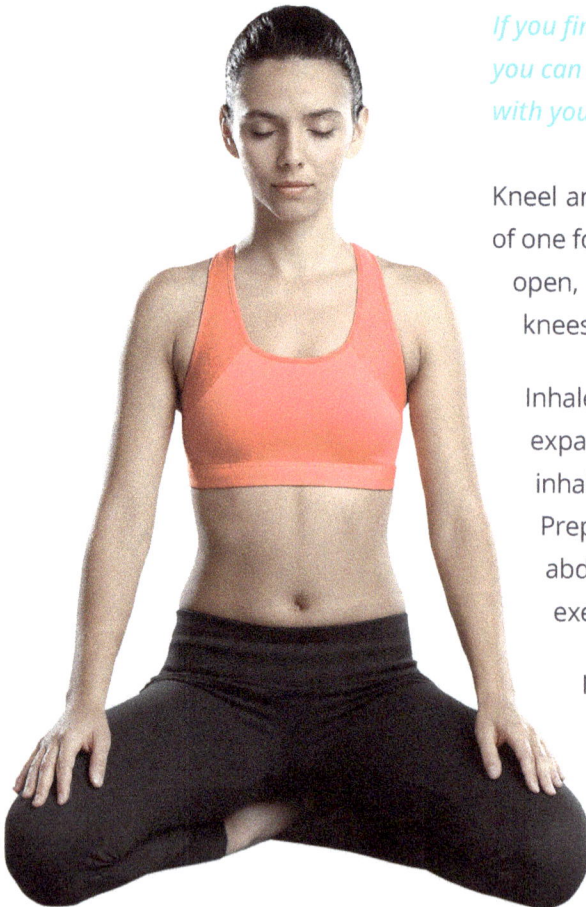

If you find it difficult to sit on the floor, you can do this exercise sitting on a chair with your back straight.

Kneel and sit on your feet, with the toes of one foot on top of the other, the knees open, and your hands resting on the knees or thighs.

Inhale and exhale a couple of times, expanding your abdomen on the inhalation as much as possible. Preparing the expansion of the abdomen in this way makes the exercise more effective.

Inhale and exhale smoothly and fluidly, but also with intent, with presence, expanding fully but gently on the inhalation and emptying thoroughly on the exhalation.

Having inhaled and exhaled thoroughly a few times, firmly place the palms of your hands on the lower ribs toward the back, resting the lower ridge of your palms on the crest of your hips.

Keep the hands controlled and engaged with the fingers pointing straight out in front, and press in the lower ribs with your palms. Do it with a certain intent, with presence and control – not too strongly, but firmly.

Inhale deeply and let the air move from the abdomen upward.

Because of the position, even if you try, you will not be able to bloat the abdomen. The expansion is naturally controlled, limited, and shaped. Only the upper part of the abdomen will expand. The expansion will continue upward toward the chest, giving you a clear understanding of how to start to correctly train the first phase of complete breathing.

At this point, without pausing, blocking, or tensing, exhale smoothly and fully.

Then, keeping the controlled pressure of your hands on the lower ribs, inhale again. The exercise will not work unless you keep firm control of the sides with the pressure of your hands.

Repeat this exercise three times, then stop; put your hands on the knees, relax, and observe the effect of the exercise on the position and the breathing.

Remember to always keep the back well aligned.

After practicing the exercise in this way, you can also repeat it with a pause after the exhalation. Holding the breath out, briefly stay empty and then let the inhalation start to expand.

Repeat this alternate version of the exercise one to three times, then relax and observe how it has influenced and modified your breathing experience.

If you find it helpful in the beginning, you can also start the exercise with your chin tucked against the chest so as to experience full abdominal breathing. After two or three rounds of breathing, you can untuck the chin as soon as you start the upward movement of the inhalation – and then tuck it again toward the end of exhalation.

EXERCISE 2: BOTTOM-UP LATERAL EXPANSION

👎 CHALLENGING

The second intercostal exercise trains the lateral and upward expansion of the breathing. Using the metaphor described earlier, here the emphasis of the direction of the breath is on the two sides of the arrowhead shape.

The effect is achieved by firmly and actively squeezing the abdomen during exhalation by pressing your hands into your sides, thumbs to the back, while your fingers press into the navel.

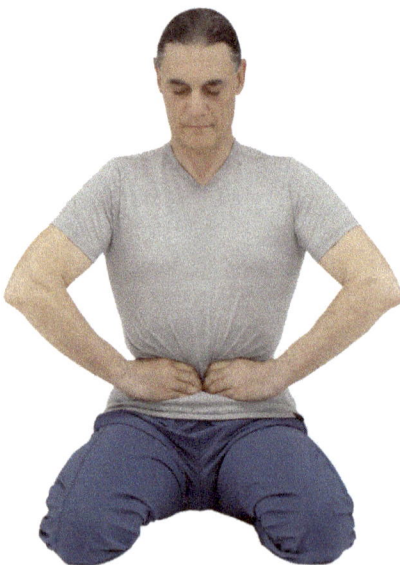

There are three ways to perform this exercise:

The first is to keep squeezing while inhaling. The inhalation will be limited and a bit difficult, but it will start to open the sides. This is also a preparation for the two main versions of the exercise.

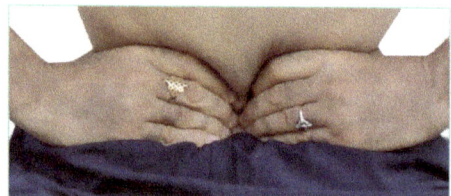

The second and most effective way is to start inhaling while just for a moment releasing the strong squeeze on your navel. Then, immediately after the brief release, block the squeeze of the navel again, keeping a firm, tight control – and in this way continue to complete the inhalation with an expansion of the sides.

If you have any difficulty applying the main exercise described above, you can use this alternative:

After thoroughly exhaling and manually contracting the abdominal muscles by strongly squeezing your navel area, hold empty for a moment. While empty, release the strong control of the abdomen just a little – very little – then immediately lock again in this new position with a firm hold on the sides of the abdomen, and inhale as fully as you can.

Incorporating a moment of empty hold will make your experience easier and clearer.

Regardless which version you choose, do not repeat this exercise more than five times in a session.

To conclude, relax in the position and observe the effect of the exercise on your breathing pattern. Keep the back straight and be mindful of your respiration. It is worth repeating that here, too, we always breathe through the nostrils and not the mouth.

In doing these exercises we learn how to expand correctly and train our capacity to breathe without blocking or fragmenting the upward flow of the inhalation.

EXPERIENCING YOUR DORSAL BREATHING CAPACITY

The dorsal breathing exercises help mobilize the rib cage and open up the diaphragm. They also help increase the overall expansion in the chest and upper chest.

Expanding the dorsal breathing capacity is especially beneficial for people who have a contracted, blocked diaphragm and a habit of shallow breathing.

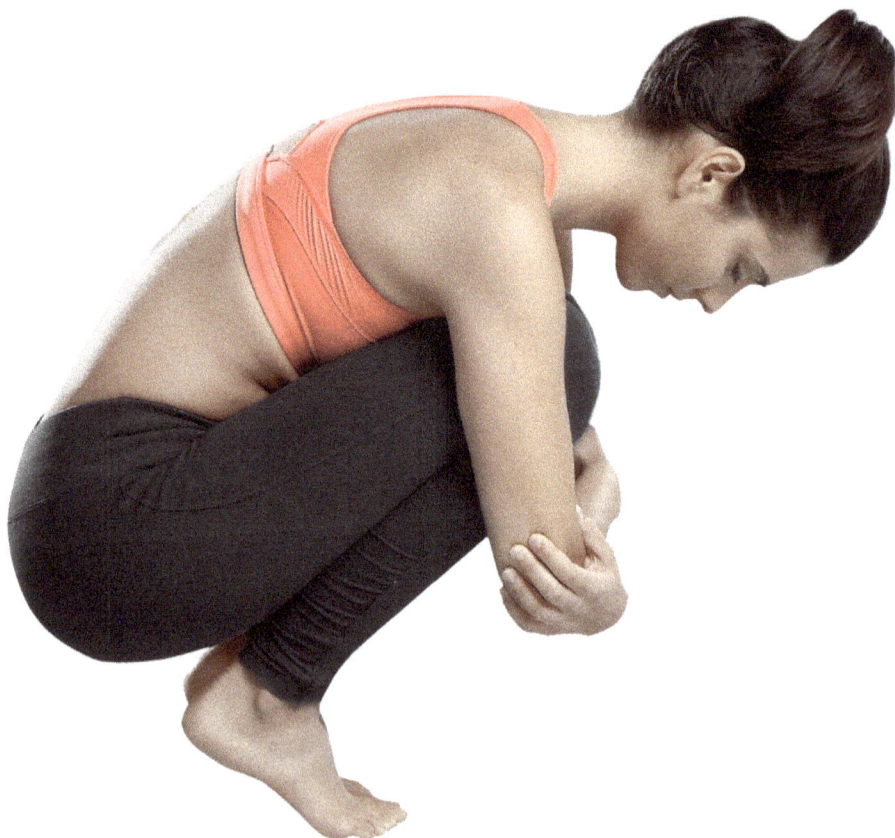

EXERCISE 1: KNEE-HUGGING SQUAT

👍 EASY

This exercise for improving dorsal breathing is done by balancing on your feet and hugging your knees firmly while breathing deeply in the abdomen.

If it is more comfortable, you can put a prop or a pillow under your heels or buttocks.

Inhale and exhale deeply but smoothly a few times. Observe closely the experience of expansion and opening in the back.

If you use props, be sure to lean forward, otherwise you will lose the experience of the lower dorsal expansion. Keeping a forward inclination will facilitate the dorsal expansion in the lower or middle part of the torso.

As with all these exercises, do your best to breathe deeply into the abdomen because the abdominal phase is the base, the foundation of perfect breathing.

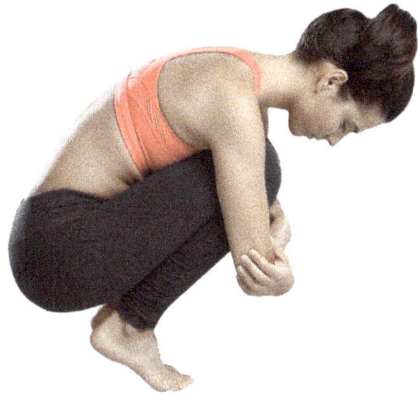

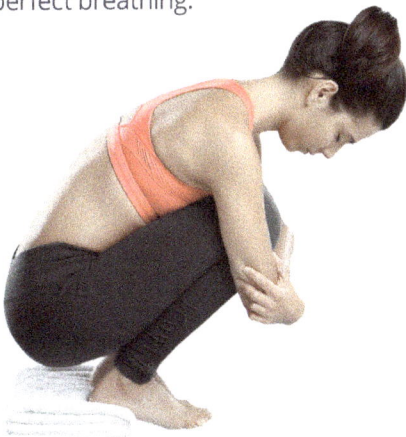

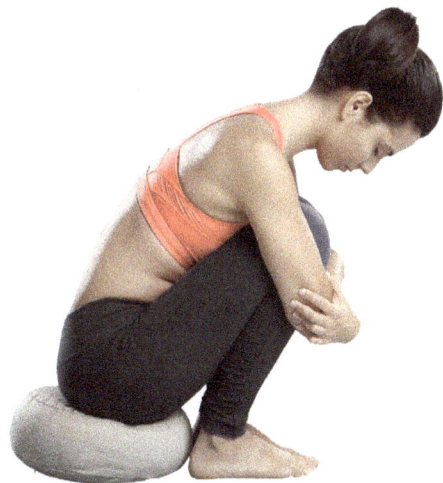

EXERCISE 2: SIMPLIFIED DORSAL TRAINING

👍 EASY

The second exercise is another way to experience dorsal breathing. It is also a useful alternative if you find the Knee-Hugging Squat difficult. This is the same as the simple exercise introduced in the beginning of this part of the book.

Simply kneel with your knees together, bend forward, place your elbows on the floor in front of your knees, and cradle your head in the palms of your hands. Then breathe deeply and fully.

Alternatively, sit on a chair with your knees together and place the elbows on the thighs, just above the knees.

This position allows an experience of the central range of dorsal breathing. Breathe from below, deeply and fluidly.

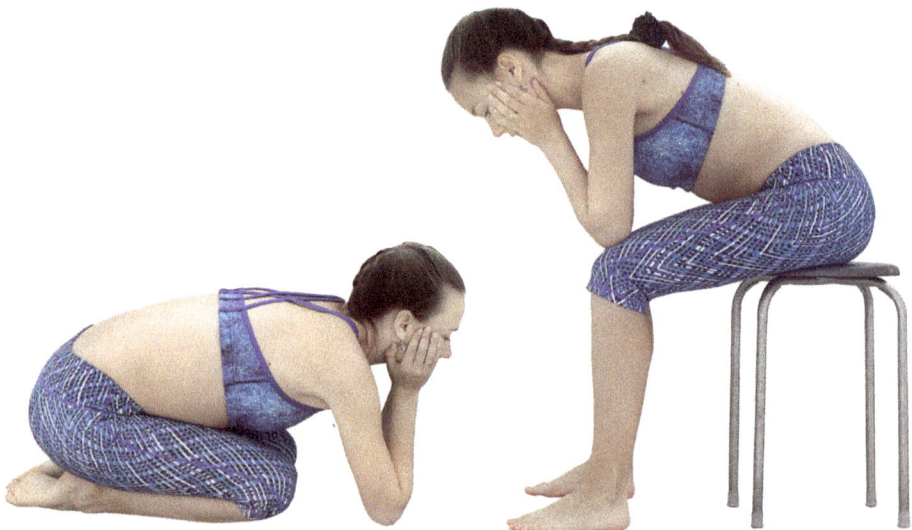

DEVELOPING THE THORACIC PHASE

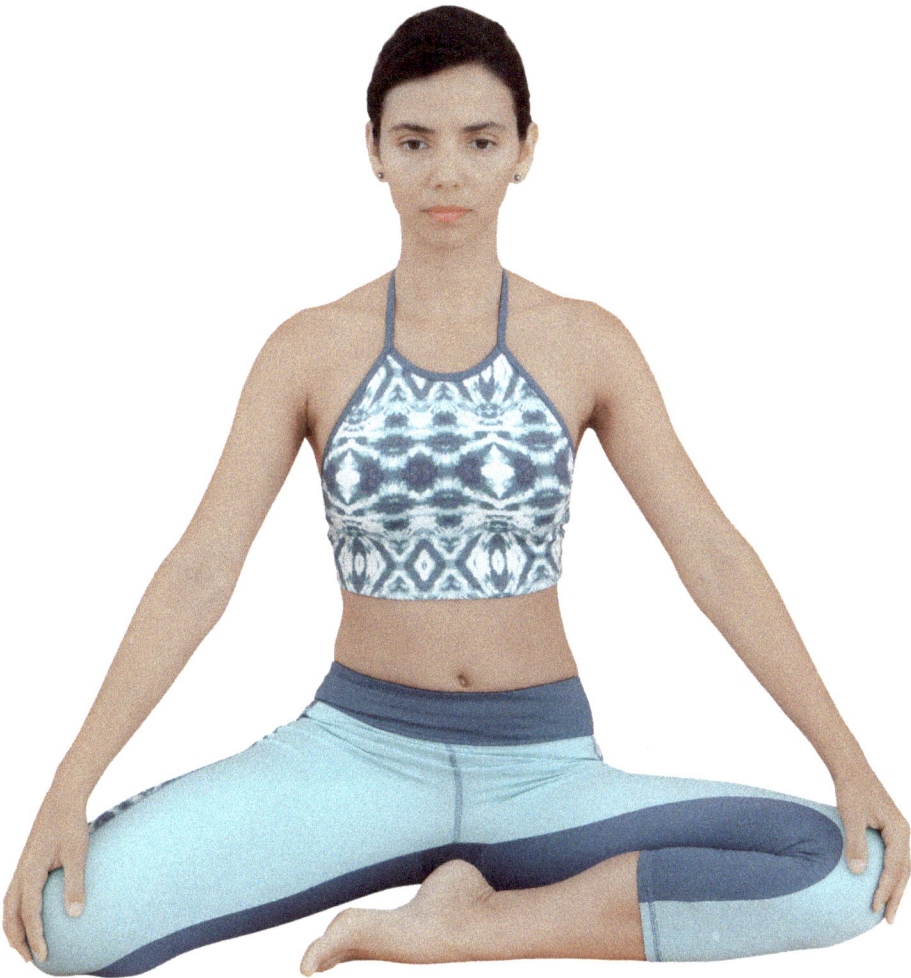

| n these exercises the air expands mostly into the upper part of the lungs, physically opening the chest and allowing for full upper-chest breathing.

EXERCISE 1: CHEST OPENER

👍 EASY

The first thoracic phase exercise helps open and expand the chest and can be done with or without props.

Performing this exercise without props is bit challenging unless you have at least some degree of flexibility and experience. It therefore makes sense in this case to present the supported version first.

You can use one or more pillows or blankets as props, setting them up in a way that will allow a gentle arch of your lower back, but with the top your head lower than the shoulders. Gently lie down on your props, with your legs stretched out straight, and breathe deeply through the nostrils into the chest.

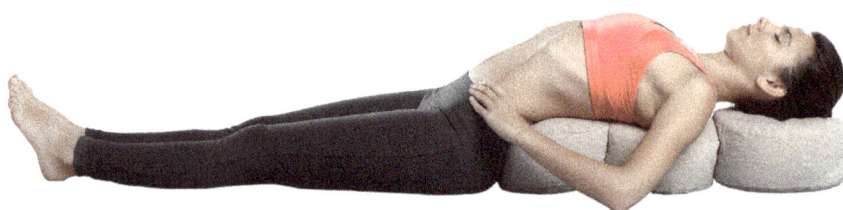

If you are not comfortable with your head lower than your chest, change the setup of the props so your head is supported at the same level as the shoulders. Breathe and relax, deeply focusing your awareness mostly in the chest.

For an even gentler and easier variation, rearrange the props to support the head a little higher than before. The main point is to genuinely feel comfortable so that you can focus all your attention on fully expanding the breath and in particular on the expansion of the chest.

The less you arch your back in this last position, the harder it will be to focus mostly on the expansion in the chest. It is quite possible you will also note an expansion in the abdomen, but this is fine as long as the chest expansion is happening.

UNSUPPORTED VERSION

 CHALLENGING

If you feel comfortable practicing without props, lie on the floor with your legs close together. Supporting yourself on your elbows, lift your torso up as you arch back and place the top of your head on the ground.

Bring your hands to your sides, fingers forward, and thumbs back. This will help you open the shoulders.

Breathe and try to expand your respiration well within the chest.

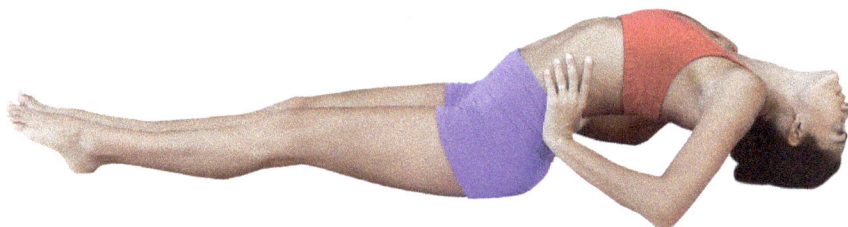

When you come out of the position, carefully ease the head back to the floor and then turn to one side before rising up to sitting.

EXERCISE 2: ACTIVE UPPER CHEST OPENER

👆 CHALLENGING

This exercise serves to actively open and train the upper chest breathing. It may be a little challenging, so take care to try it out gently and with awareness. It is best to prepare for it with some dedicated warm-ups (such as the Snake Training exercises). You can also easily substitute it with one or more of the subsequent exercises.

Lie with your legs close together, forehead on the ground, and hands under the shoulders, palms flat on the floor. Gently arch your upper torso, coming to rest on your elbows, forearms, and hands and keeping the legs and feet together.

Remaining in the position without lifting the base of the thighs off the floor, when exhaling, move your shoulders forward, closing and squeezing the upper chest. When inhaling, rotate the shoulders back and open the upper chest. The head remains straight; the only movement is in the shoulders and chest. Repeat a few times.

EXERCISE 3: FORWARD-RESTING CHEST OPENER I

 CHALLENGING

This next exercise can be easier. It is also more passive. Ideally, you can prepare for it with the corresponding warm-up (Turn and Stretch).

As in the Turn and Stretch warm-up, start by sitting on the floor with one leg bent in front and the heel at the perineum. Bend the other leg behind you, keeping the foot close to your buttocks without sitting on it.

Bend forward to place the side of the head and, if possible, the shoulders on the ground. Turn your head to the side you find more comfortable, but keep it centered between the knees.

As you bend forward, keep the buttocks as close as possible to the floor. If this proves uncomfortable, try one of the variations described below or substitute with the next exercise.

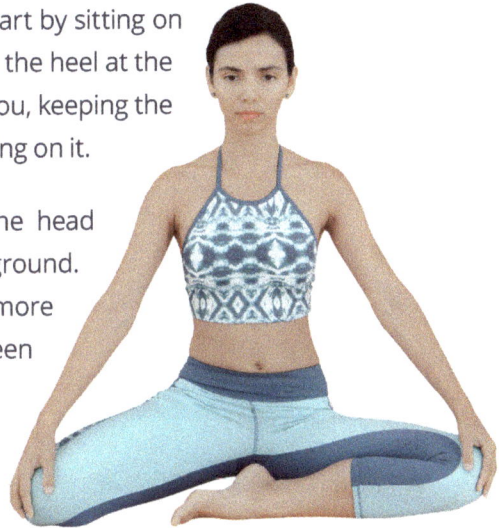

Alternate calm, relaxed breathing with a more active, intentional expansion on the inhalation. Apply this principle to all of the following exercises.

After a few rounds of breath, reverse the position of the legs and the head and repeat as before.

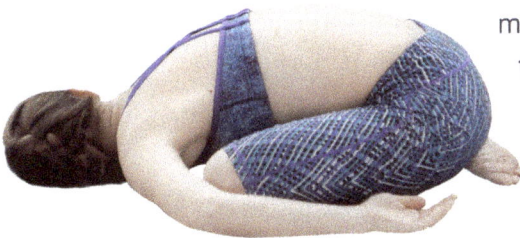

If you find it too uncomfortable, you can rest your forehead on the ground, on your fists, on your hands, or on your crossed arms. However, in this case, to maintain the dynamics of the exercise, it is advisable that you also lift your buttocks a bit by sitting on a cushion between your legs. Additionally, you may find it helpful to place some firm cushions under your shoulders. Examples of all these adaptations are shown for the next exercise.

👍 MODERATE

Here is yet another position for "passively" opening your upper chest breathing. It is also an easier option if the previous exercise is too challenging or too difficult to perform.

Sit on your heels with your knees open, one foot on top of the other or one next to the other. If needed you can put a pillow under your buttocks to make the position more comfortable.

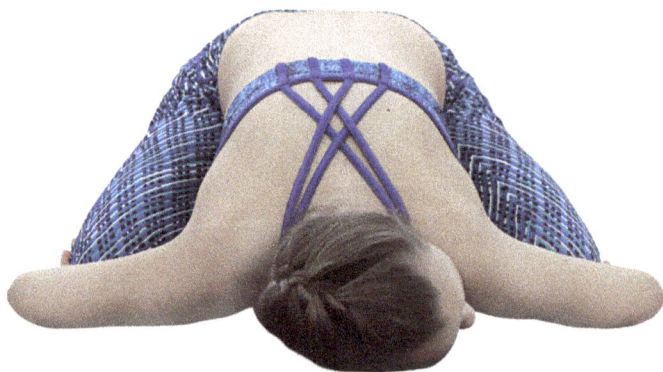

Bend forward and rest the side of your face on the floor. Breathe and relax, feeling how the upper chest opens and expands. Alternate with some deep inhalations.

Then change the position of the head to face the other side and breathe a few times, alternating calm, relaxed breathing with a more active, intentional expansion on the inhalation.

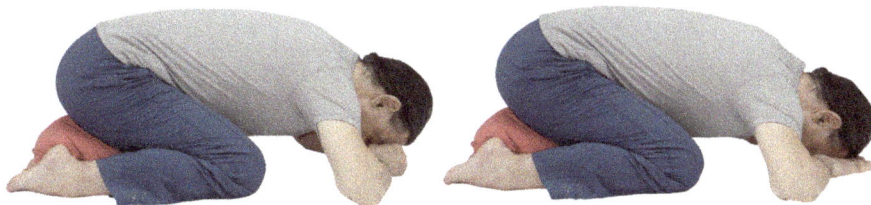

ALTERNATE VERSION

👍 EASY

For an easier version, you can also rest your forehead on the ground, on your fists, on your hands, or on your crossed arms, but in this case it is better to have a cushion under your buttocks as well.

In many positions where you rest your head on the ground in front of you, having the shoulders supported allows for a better, more precise experience. For this reason, if needed, you can place a pillow, a folded blanket, or any other useful prop under each shoulder for support.

As in the previous exercise, you can also put props such as firm pillows under your shoulders to help you relax into the position and focus your attention entirely on the correct application of the breathing.

You can achieve the same effect seated on a chair:

Sitting near the edge of a chair, bend forward and take hold of your ankles or leave your crossed arms on your knees.

Rest in the position and alternate soft breathing with deep inhalations.

RELAX, OPEN, AND DISCOVER

EXERCISE 1: SUPINE TWIST

👍 EASY

This exercise is highly effective for teaching yourself to open up to a more complete breathing. In doing so, you will also achieve more flexibility. You can use the expansion of the breathing to open up and release tensions in the body from the inside out. It is also an important exercise for discovering and developing awareness of your respiration. Like all Harmonious Breathing exercises, the inhalation starts from below, in the abdomen.

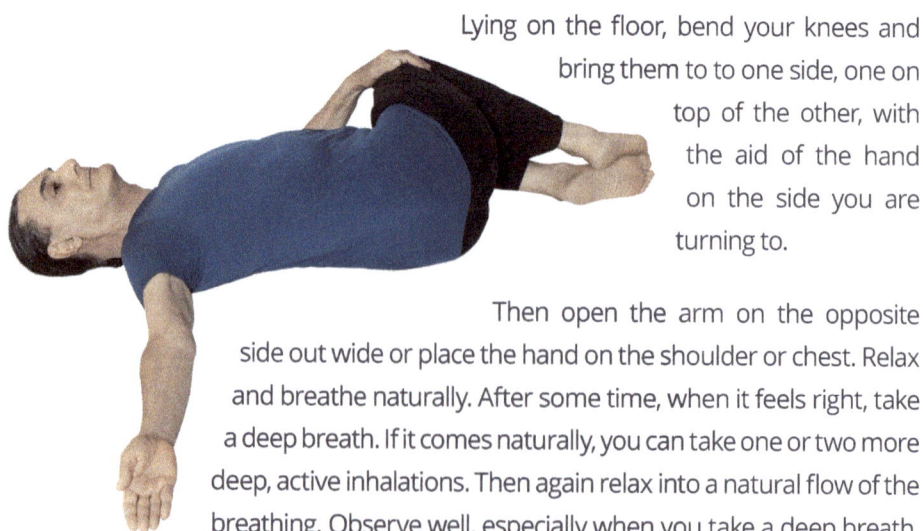

Lying on the floor, bend your knees and bring them to to one side, one on top of the other, with the aid of the hand on the side you are turning to.

Then open the arm on the opposite side out wide or place the hand on the shoulder or chest. Relax and breathe naturally. After some time, when it feels right, take a deep breath. If it comes naturally, you can take one or two more deep, active inhalations. Then again relax into a natural flow of the breathing. Observe well, especially when you take a deep breath, and you will experience an expansion of the abdomen, the side at the intercostal level, and in the back (the dorsal area).

In particular, you will feel your breathing opening and expanding in the upper abdomen, especially toward the open side.

Alternating deep breathing with more natural breathing will keep your experience relaxed and fresh.

Then roll onto the other side and repeat.

Afterward, you can relax with your back straight and experience how smooth, fluid, and complete your respiration has become.

This exercise can also be used to experience how movement and position can influence the degree and dynamics of the breathing. By simply moving your arm up or down you can discover how this influences the pattern of the respiration.

By leaving your arm down along the side, you will not feel as much of a side and back expansion, but more of a chest expansion.

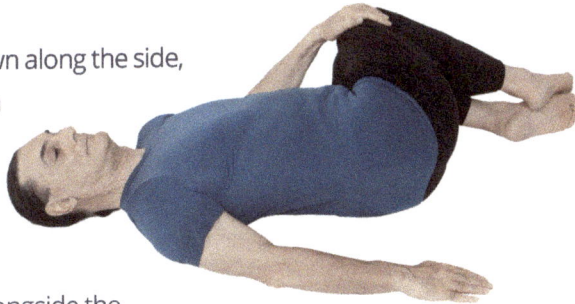

Bringing your arm up alongside the head will provide a clearer focus on the chest and upper torso breathing, including a dorsal expansion.

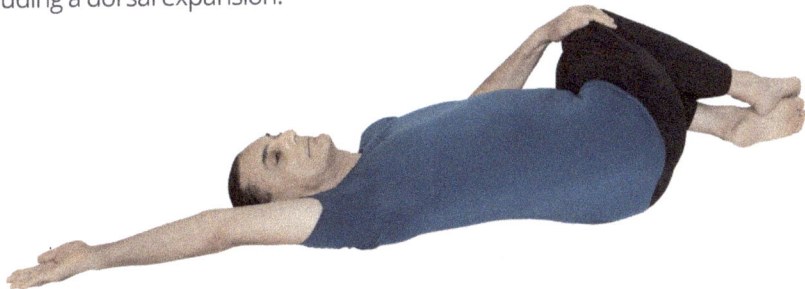

EXERCISE 2: RESTING DOVE

👍 MODERATE

This position is particularly useful for experiencing and training the abdominal and lateral dorsal expansion in "bottom-up" inhalation. Also, it is another useful tool for discovering and exploring a relaxed and open quality in your respiration.

Lie on your stomach with your head turned to one side and bring the knee of the leg on that side up toward the shoulder. Keeping the shoulders on the floor, rest both arms along the sides, or, if you find it more comfortable, place your elbow against the raised knee with your arm on the floor.

You can use a small cushion under your lower rib cage or under your head and can also bring the back arm under your head for support.

Rest and breathe in a relaxed way, without intentionally controlling your breathing. When it feels right, take a deep inhalation and observe how and where the breath expands. Then again relax the breathing.

Alternate between relaxed and deeper breathing for a while.

You can also experiment with a relaxed, passive pause at the bottom of the exhalation, briefly staying empty of breath before inhaling again.

Then turn to the other side and repeat the exercise.

THE FOUR KEYS TO COMPLETE BREATHING

While the exercises we have covered so far provide a comprehensive experience of complete breathing, in Harmonious Breathing we also teach what we call the Four Keys. These exercises can easily be done by most people, even without any particular training. They serve as a helpful tool for sequentially and correctly unlocking, opening, and connecting the four main phases of complete breathing: from abdominal to intercostal (First Key), intercostal to chest (Second Key), and chest to upper chest (Third Key). The Fourth Key works on further expanding upper chest breathing.

They can be performed kneeling, in any stable sitting position, or even standing, as long as the spine is firm and straight. As in the previous exercises, the inhalations are always from the bottom up, while the exhalations are from the top down.

What makes the Four Keys so useful is that simply by doing them, we successively and harmoniously develop our capacity for complete breathing.

They can serve as a stand-alone set in a quick and easy session or compliment any of the other exercises. You can do all four or just whichever one is most relevant for the aspect of the breathing you are focusing on.

When applied in sequence, after each exercise and the period following each for observing its effects, move the arms into position to continue with the next exercise.

The exercises are meant to be performed with intent and strength, both in the movement and breathing. All breathing is through the nostrils – fluid and with vigor.

When you have more confidence you can explore the difference between doing these exercises with faster movements and more vigorous breathing and with slower, calmer, smoother breathing.

You can also do them in a continuous, vigorous sequence, merging the final exhalation of one exercise directly with the first inhalation of the next.

However, overdoing any kind of exercise can cause the volume of carbon dioxide ventilated to exceed the body's production of it, and this, in turn, leads to hyperventilation. Many people equate hyperventilation with rapid, shallow breathing, but in fact it is just as much linked with excessive deep breathing, or "overbreathing." So you should be aware that excessive exercise – regardless of pace – can exaggerate your air element.

> With all of these exercises, it is important to bear in mind that overdoing breathwork can disproportionately intensify the air element within our system. The air element is related to movement, to lightness. If the air element is too strong, we may experience some imbalance, especially late in the evening. This is why you might find it difficult to fall asleep if you practice too much, too vigorously, or too late in the day.
>
> Later in life, we need to take special care not to aggravate the air element since it already tends to be more predominant at this stage.
>
> With this in mind, do not overdo it. Do not force. Do not practice late in the evening.

THE FIRST KEY: ABDOMINAL TO INTERCOSTAL

👍 EASY

All Four Keys work with abdominal breathing as the foundation, while the position and rotations of the arms and shoulders are used to shape the breathing.

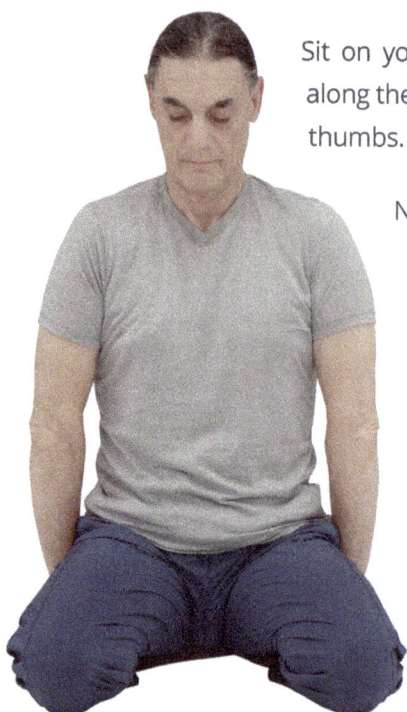

Sit on your heels, knees apart, back straight, arms along the sides, and hands closed in a fist around the thumbs. Inhale.

Now exhale, rotating the shoulders and arms forward to close the shoulders and squeeze the chest and abdomen.

Keep your back aligned and stable in this process. The movement should be vigorous, but the breathing calm and yet with intent.

Inhale, focusing on expanding the abdomen while rotating the shoulders back and bringing your shoulder blades toward each other.

Exhale, rotating the shoulders forward and closing the chest. Inhale, rotating them back and opening the chest.

After a sequence of no more than three to five rounds of respiration, stop, place your hands on your knees, and observe your breathing.

Do not try to change or decide anything, just observe and experience. Notice if and how the exercise has changed the dynamics of your respiration.

After a few relaxed rounds of breathing in this way, you can repeat the exercise once more, this time introducing a brief pause after the exhalation. The pause, or "empty hold," could be two counts, or two slow seconds, but no longer than that.

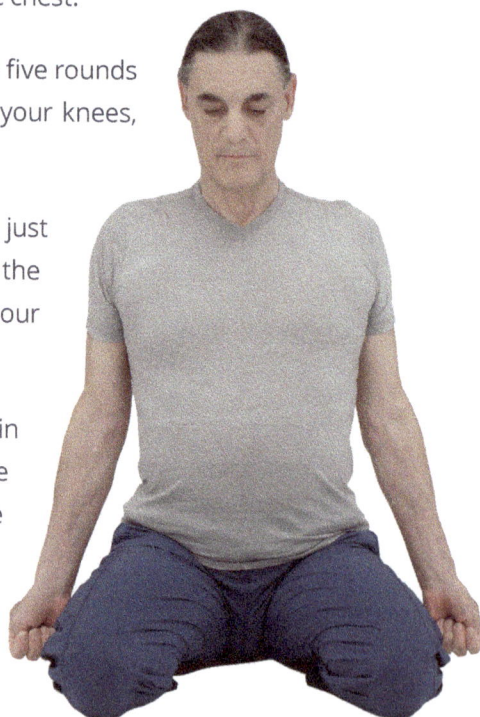

Whenever we add a moment of empty hold after the exhalation, we will notice how it increases the expansion of the breathing. It also makes us more aware of how the inhalation can and should start in the abdomen, and how this is the root of harmonious, natural breathing. But here, too, it is important not to overdo it.

With this in mind, it is best not to repeat the exercise more than three or four times in a single session. To conclude, rest with your hands on your knees.

When applied in a routine or sequence, you can choose which way you want to practice it; even one repetition could be enough.

Be aware how the breathing occurs and relax into it, without wanting to change it or shape it, just observing and experiencing.

You will notice that very gradually the breathing starts to contract again. This is our habit, our body memory that starts to recondition our breathing. It is completely normal, but this is precisely why we have to train, to change the body's memory. By acquiring a new memory we decondition our habitual breathing and allow it to find a more natural and free condition.

In the beginning, it can also be helpful to start the exercise with your chin tucked in toward or against the chest, lifting it soon after you start the inhalation, then closing it again at the end of exhalation.

If you feel tired you can straighten out the legs, relax, and gently move and shake your legs and arms.

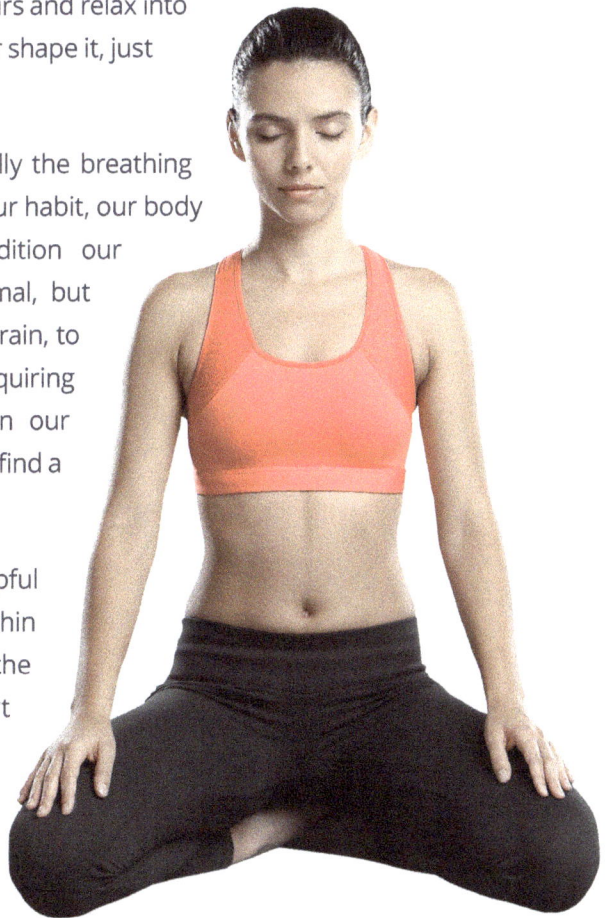

THE SECOND KEY: INTERCOSTAL TO CHEST

👍 EASY

The Second Key repeats a similar sequence of movements, but with your arms a bit more out to the side.

To gauge the distance, you should still be able to touch the tips of your fingers to the ground with the arms open.

The rotational movement of shoulders and arms is the same as in the First Key, but this time the movement is designed to train the intercostal breathing, which opens primarily into the lower part of the rib cage.

Exhale well, then inhale, focusing on expanding the abdomen. At the same time, with intent and presence, rotate your shoulders and arms back. As your shoulder blades move toward each other, you should feel the lower rib cage opening and expanding.

Exhale, rotating the arms and shoulders forward to contract the rib cage and squeeze the air out.

Inhale, focusing on expanding from below, while rotating your arms and shoulders back to open the intercostal breathing.

After a sequence of no more than three to five rounds of breath, stop, put your hands on your knees, and without controlling or modifying it observe how the breathing manifests.

Notice if and how the exercise has changed the dynamics of your respiration.

After a few rounds of relaxed breathing, repeat the exercise, this time with a brief pause after the exhalation. The pause or empty hold could be two counts, or two slow seconds, but no more than that.

Repeat the exercise with an empty pause, but no more than one to three times. Then let the breathing be. Do not try to change or shape it. Just observe.

THE THIRD KEY: CHEST TO UPPER CHEST

👍 EASY

The Third Key consists of repeating a similar sequence of movements, but this time with your arms open wide to the side. The hands can either be closed in a fist or open, but firmly controlled.

Start by exhaling fully. Then inhale, focusing on starting from below, while rotating your arms and shoulders back to open the chest wide, vigorously breaking through blockages and tensions.

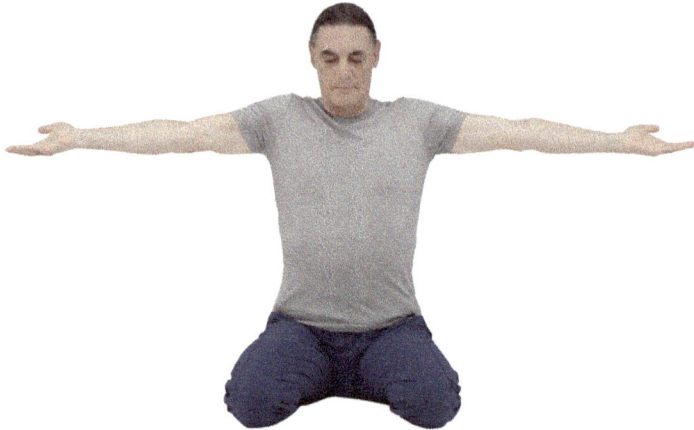

Exhale, rotating the shoulders forward, contracting and thoroughly emptying the upper chest and chest. Then inhale once more, again rotating your arms and shoulders back to open the chest wide.

After a sequence of no more than three to five rounds of breathing, stop, put your hands on your knees, and observe the movement of the breathing. Notice if and how the exercise has changed the dynamics of your respiration.

After a few rounds of breathing in this way, repeat the exercise with a brief empty pause after the exhalation, for a total of one, two, or at most three more rounds.

Now place your hands on your knees. Observe your breathing. Notice if and how the exercise has changed the dynamics of your respiration.

THE FOURTH KEY: COLLARBONE

👍 EASY

The Fourth Key focuses more precisely on expanding into the top of your lungs, with a sensation of bringing the breath into the clavicular or collarbone region.

Sit on your heels with your knees open and hands behind your back, fingers interlocked. As always, remember to keep the back aligned and controlled.

Throughout this exercise, keep your back stable, neither bent forward nor arched backward, and your palms facing up.

The only slight modifications in the alignment are a result of the rotation of the arms and shoulders.

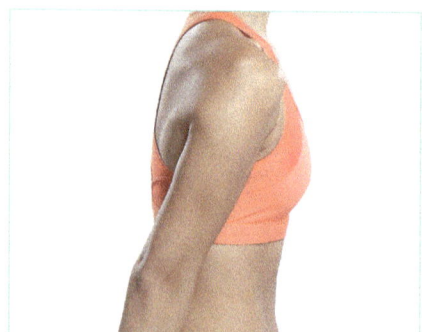

After exhaling fully, inhale and move your interlocked fingers backward and downward while vigorously pulling your shoulders back to open the upper chest and expand the breathing.

Exhaling, rotate the shoulders forward, contracting, squeezing and thoroughly emptying the area from the upper chest to the abdomen.

Inhale, again rotating the shoulders back to open the chest and upper chest.

After a sequence of three to five rounds of breathing, stop, put your hands on your knees, and for a few respirations observe the movement of the breathing, its new dynamics, without wanting to influence or act on the experience.

Now repeat the exercise, this time with a brief pause in empty hold after the exhalation, at most one to three more times.

Place your hands on your knees and enjoy the new expansiveness of your breathing, an expansiveness that breaks through tensions and just happens by itself, beyond intention.

Just observe and experience.

ALTERNATIVE VERSIONS

The Four Keys can also be done sitting on a chair, or even standing.

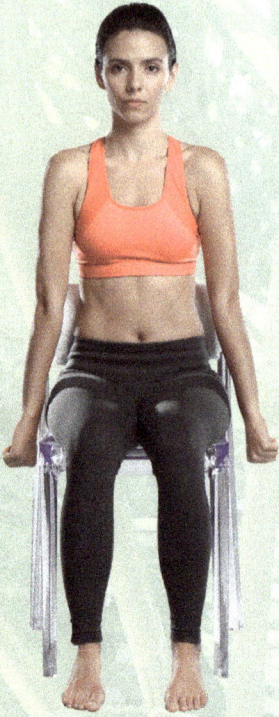

For the chair version, simply sit near the edge of a chair, with the feet placed firmly on the ground and the spine correctly aligned.

If you need a support to keep the back straight, roll a towel and place it behind you, in the small of your back. Adjust the thickness of the towel to allow you to have the back properly aligned. To avoid creating tension in the abdomen and impairing the expansion of the breathing, arch the lower back only to the extent that comes naturally.

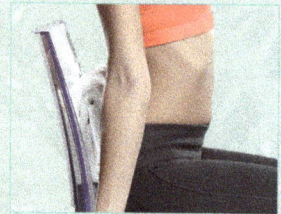

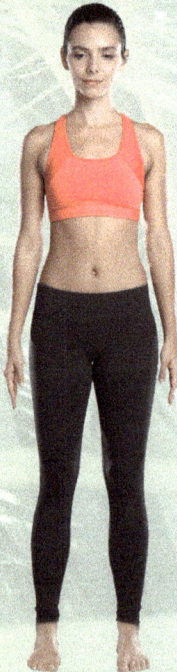

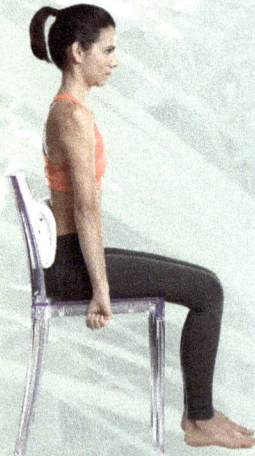

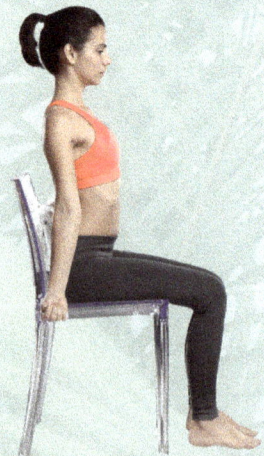

If doing the Four Keys standing, make sure that your position is balanced and stable, with the back straight.

COORDINATING THE FOUR PHASES

So far, we have experienced the individual stages of complete breathing separately, focusing mainly on the inhalation. Before moving on to the next set, where we concentrate on the quality of the exhalations, each of these next four exercises is designed to sequentially coordinate the four stages of breathing into a single, harmonious, flowing, and smooth upward movement.

EXERCISE 1: INHALING SLOWLY

👍 EASY

This exercise is a basic practice in Yantra Yoga and is the first of what we call the Eight Movements to Purify the Prana.

Like most sequences in Yantra Yoga, it is meant to be performed with a specific breathing rhythm. Each phase is done in two counts of a little more than a second each, except for the central long inhalation, which is done in four counts.

Stand straight, with your feet and legs parallel and your arms at your sides.

Inhaling in two counts, grasp each arm with the other hand just above the elbow, slightly pressing each arm with your thumbs. Raise your arms to shoulder height, still within the two-count inhalation.

The movement starts on opposite sides of the body for men and women. Women first grasp the right arm with the left hand. Men first grasp of the left arm with the right hand.

Exhaling in two counts, lower your arms toward the abdomen while exhaling fully from top to bottom.

The downward movement and the position of the arms facilitate exhaling from top to bottom, ending at the abdomen.

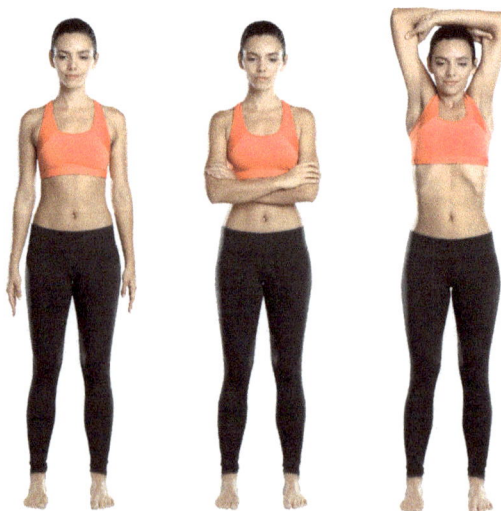

In four counts, inhale slowly and completely, starting from the abdomen, as you stretch your arms above your head and expand the air upward into the chest and upper chest. Keep your torso straight to achieve and experience a correct and complete inhalation.

When your arms reach over your head, the top of the movement, energetically tense and stretch the whole body, holding the air without blocking.

The sequence should be experienced as a continuous expansion of the chest, aided by the upward stretching of the arms, where the held air creates the sensation of expanding in an open space.

Exhale in two counts, opening your arms wide and lowering them to your sides.

Inhale in two counts as you raise your arms to a level slightly above shoulder height, opening them wide, like eagle's wings.

Exhaling in two counts, lower your arms back down along the sides.

Repeat the sequence two more times. Then remain standing for a while, observing the natural flow of your breathing.

To experience how the exercise helps coordinate your breathing, at the conclusion you can place one hand on the abdomen and the other on the chest and notice the harmonious flow of the breath.

EXERCISE 2: DOWN, UP, AND ARCH

This simple exercise can be done in three different versions to suit your flexibility: a challenging standing version and a simpler one that achieves a similar effect without requiring you to bend all the way forward and down as well as a moderate seated version.

Full Version

CHALLENGING

Stand with your arms along the sides. Be present and check that your alignment is correct.

Breathe calmly and fluidly.

Exhaling thoroughly, gradually bend forward.

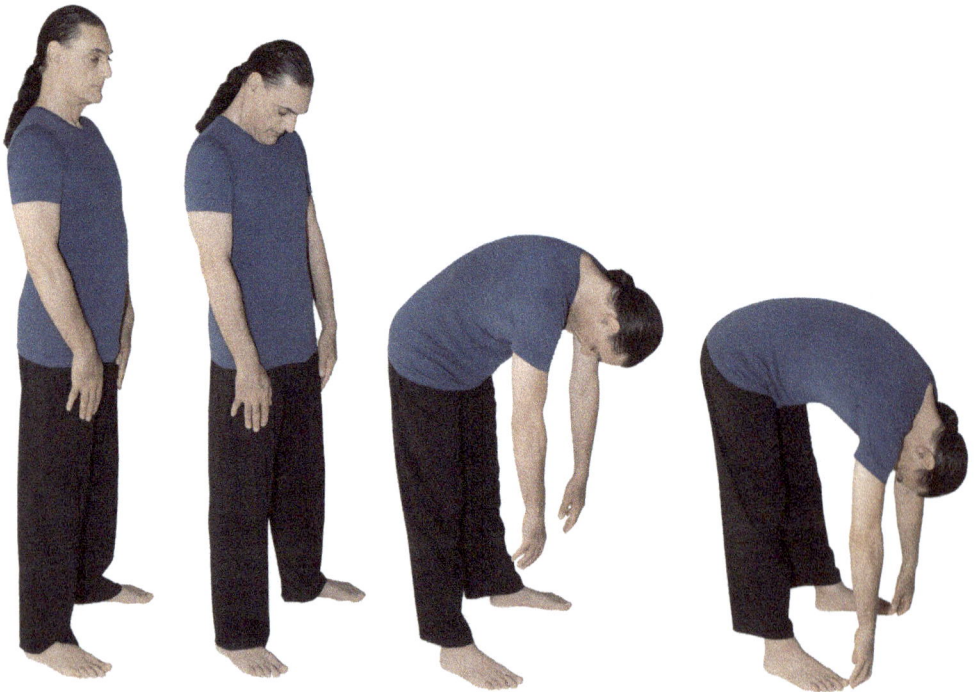

First drop the chin toward the chest, then – keeping your waist and legs controlled – bend forward toward the floor, letting go of your head and arms and releasing any tension. The legs can be either straight or slightly bent.

Now inhale as you come back up. Keeping the legs strong and waist firm, start lifting the torso, straightening from the root of the spine.

Keep rolling up until your torso and head are straight.

At this point, arch your torso backward while firmly engaging your arms and hands and opening them slightly out to the sides as you rotate the shoulders and thoroughly open the chest to a fluid, full inhalation.

Keep the waist properly engaged to avoid creating discontinuity in the movement and breathing. The movement should start at the root of the spine while the pelvis remains stable and aligned with the legs – without moving forward or caving in.

The movement of the head needs to be controlled as well. Take care not to arch too far back as it can create tension in the glottis and consequently unnecessarily strain the breathing.

From this position, without blocking the breath, smoothly transition into exhaling. Start by bringing the arms back along the sides and raising the head back to an upright position as you let the air out from the upper chest first. Then lower the chin toward the chest and start bending forward as before, continuing to exhale all the way to the bottom.

You can repeat the sequence three times; then stay in the starting position for a while, observing and following the natural flow of the breath.

Simplified Version

👍 EASY

Stand with your arms along the sides. Be present and check that your alignment is correct.

Breathe calmly and fluidly.

Exhale thoroughly as you close the chin toward the chest.

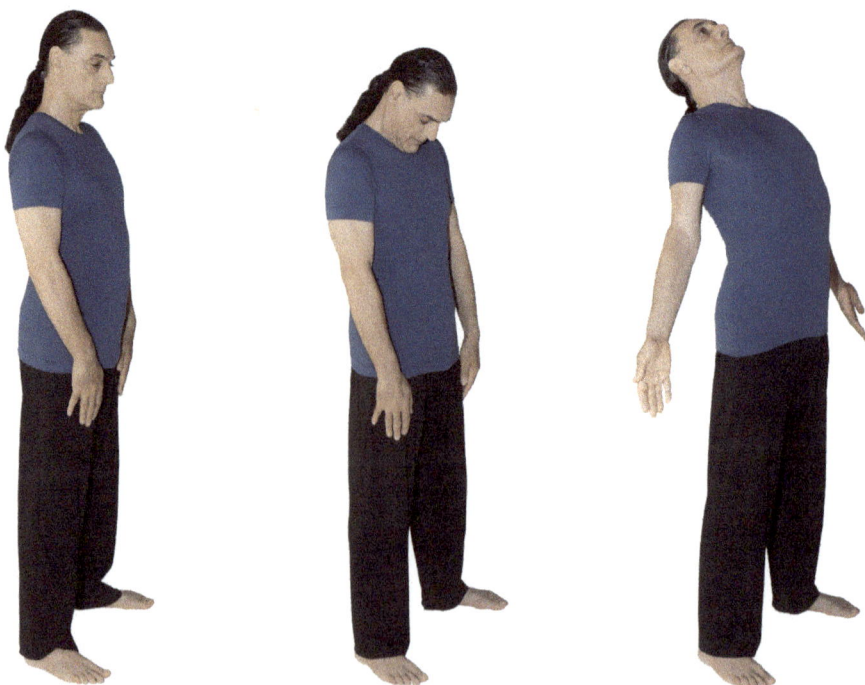

Keeping the waist and legs controlled, inhale directly from below upward, calmly and fully. Arch your torso backward from the root of the spine, vigorously opening your chest. The arms rotate and move slightly out to the sides in order to open the shoulders and the chest and allow them to complete a full inhalation.

Keeping the chin close to the chest at the start will assist you in inhaling correctly from the bottom up, expanding first in the abdomen and moving the airflow smoothly upward.

Let the upward flow of the air be what brings your body up, smoothly and effortlessly. Use the power of the inhalation to lessen the need for muscular action in your movement. Let the breathing move your body.

Now exhale as you come back to the starting position, bringing the arms back along the sides, raising the head up, and then lowering the chin toward the chest. Let the air out from the upper chest first and finish the exhalation by thoroughly emptying the abdomen.

Bringing the chin to the chest will assist you in exhaling correctly from top to bottom.

You can repeat the sequence three times; then stay in the starting position for a while, observing and following the natural flow of the breath.

Seated Version

👍 MODERATE

Sit on your heels, feet together, knees open, but not too much; you need to feel stable when arching back. Alternatively, sit on a chair with your back straight.

Let your arms hang by your sides. Breathe calmly and fluidly.

Close the chin toward the chest as you exhale thoroughly, emptying the abdomen last and contracting it toward the spine.

Keeping the pelvis firmly rooted, inhale from below, expanding the flow of breath upward while arching your torso back, rotating the arms and shoulders, and energetically opening the chest.

Now exhale to come back to the starting position, bringing the arms back along the sides and raising the head up. Continue the movement, lowering your chin and bringing it to the chest as you exhale completely.

Keep your back stable throughout the exercise.

You can repeat the sequence three to five times; then bring the hands to the knees and rest for a while in the position, observing and following the natural flow of the breath.

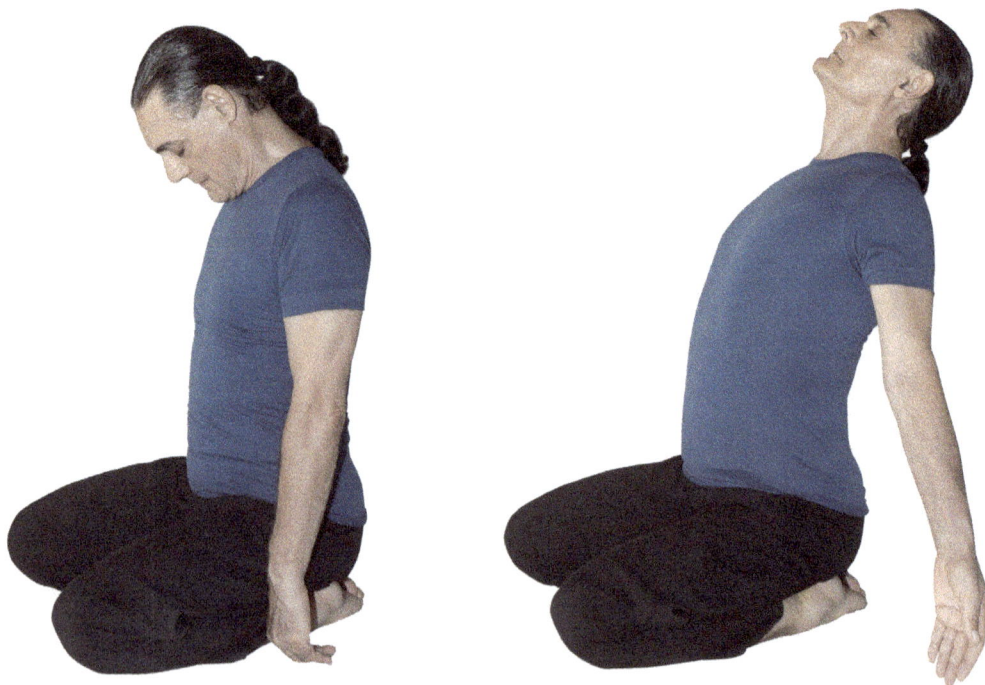

EXERCISE 3: COORDINATING CAT

👆 CHALLENGING

The third exercise in this set is another variation of the Cat. In this version, the emphasis is on coordinating a complete inhalation in a single flow of movement and breathing rather than concentrating only on the abdominal phase.

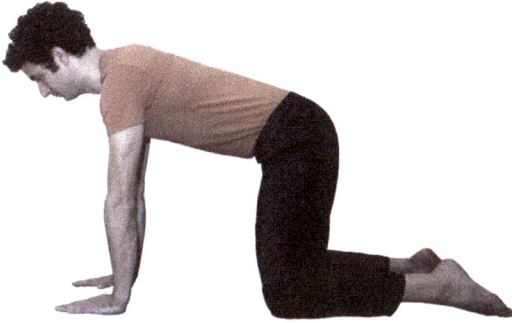

Start by coming to all fours, with your knees a shoulder width apart and arms straight. The hips should be in line with the thighs and parallel to the floor.

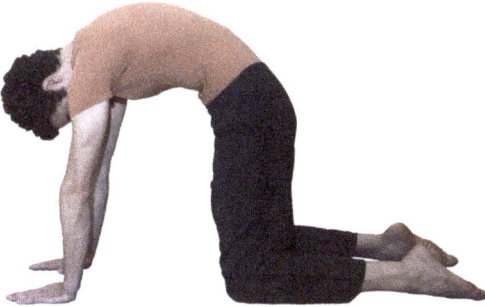

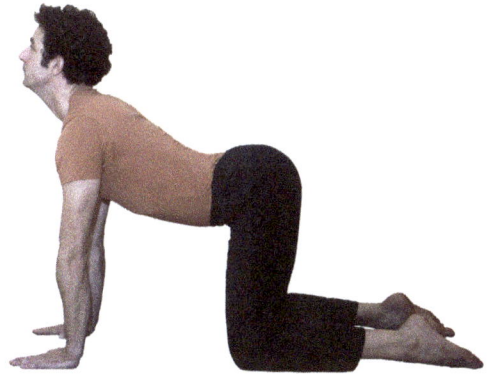

First inhale and exhale smoothly a few times.

Then, on an exhalation, bring your head between your stretched arms while rounding the mid-back, taking care to exhale thoroughly. Once empty of breath, instead of immediately inhaling, wait – holding, staying empty, while pulling the navel back toward the spine.

Wait for three counts, then release the contraction of the abdomen and let it expand fully while inhaling and counterarching the back and raising the head.

Inhale and exhale normally, then repeat the exercise for a total of at most five times.

For a more challenging variation, during the phase of the empty hold when you pull the navel toward the spine, instead of holding for only three counts, remain empty and wait until you have the natural impulse to inhale. Then release the backward pull of the abdomen, letting the inhalation start before beginning to arch the back, and only as the breath continues to expand, engage the forward and upward arching of the spine.

As mentioned in the context of the Four Keys, to minimize the possibility of hyperventilation, it is important not to overdo this exercise.

EXERCISE 4: COORDINATING BRIDGE

👍 MODERATE

This is the last of the four exercises that unite the four phases of the breathing in a single, coordinated flow. The Bridge is particularly effective in teaching you how to coordinate the individual phases of Complete Breathing and ensuring that the flow starts in the abdomen and ends in the upper chest.

The basic structure of this exercise is similar to the Bridge exercises for developing the abdominal phase as well as the one included in the warm-ups.

This version of the Bridge is a particularly good workout for the spine.

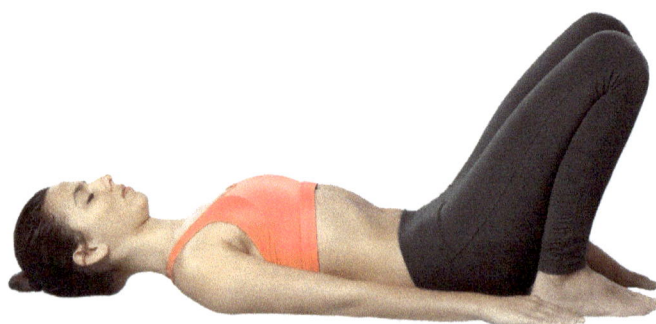

Lie on the floor with the heels close to the buttocks.

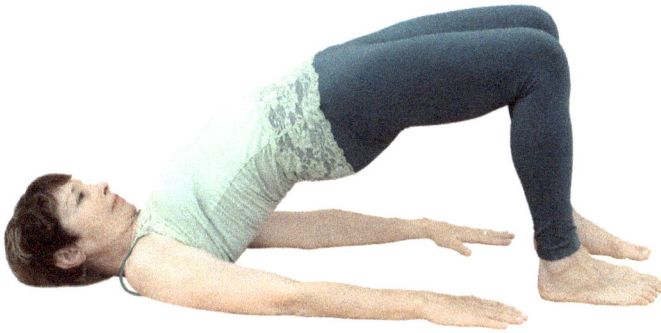

Inhale, lifting the hips and arching the back.

Exhale, bringing the hips back to the ground. Repeat the action two or three times.

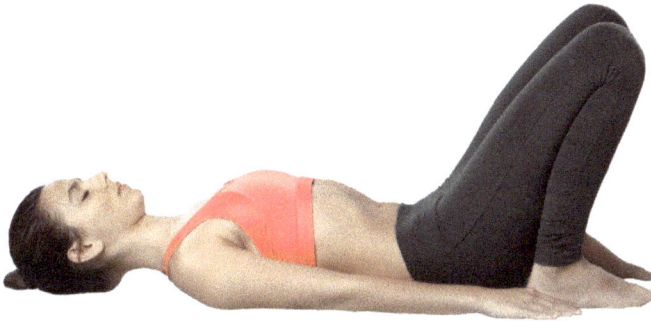

Then inhale fully while lifting the hips and arching the back. At the same time, bring the arms straight up and back to the ground, over the head, keeping them as parallel as possible.

Coordinate the sweep of the arms and the rise of the back with the gradual expansion of the inhalation.

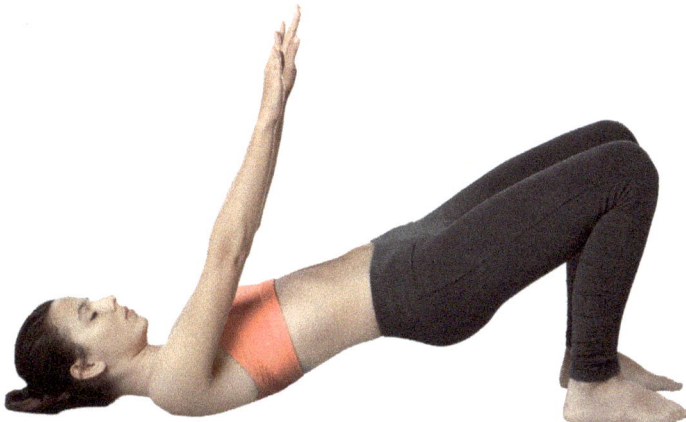

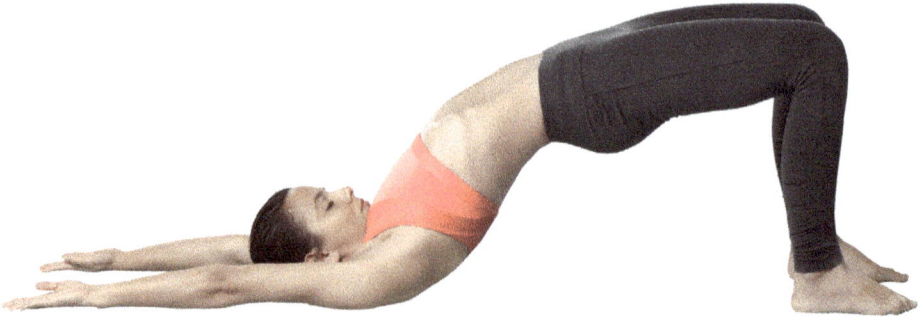

At the top of the inhalation, do not block or hold the breath. To achieve this easily, keep stretching the arms a little more along the ground, further away from the head.

In a continuous flow without pausing, exhale smoothly as you let the spine gradually come back to the floor, simultaneously bringing the arms up and down along the sides.

When you complete the exhalation, pause and remain empty for two long counts. Without moving, inhale first into the abdomen for one count and then continue to inhale while arching back up, expanding the flow of the breathing all the way up to the chest and again bringing the arms overhead.

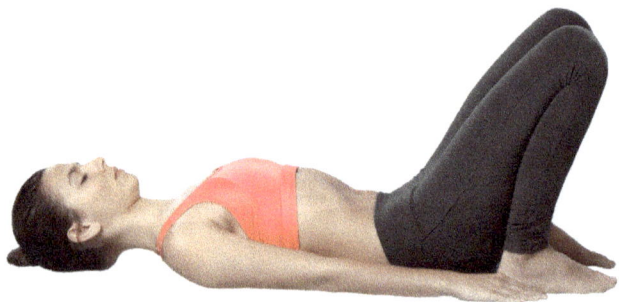

Exhale as you lower the spine back to the floor.

You can repeat this exercise as many times as you like. It is also a helpful workout for your spine.

If you feel any strain in the flow of the breath, rest with your back on the ground and take a couple of relaxed rounds of breath. Observe and discover. Then start again.

When you are familiar with the dynamics of the abdomen-first inhalation, you can stop using the empty-hold phase, keeping the focus instead on a very thorough exhalation. Repeat the basic exercise a few times, but with more focus and precise coordination.

EXHALING FROM TOP TO BOTTOM

Correct exhalation is as important as correct inhalation. The two phases are completely interdependent and ideally flow seamlessly into each other. To inhale well you need to exhale well.

Many different exhalation dynamics can be considered correct, depending how they are defined according to a given breathing technique or yoga tradition.

In Harmonious Breathing, however, the fundamental characteristic is to experience and apply a top-to-bottom exhalation, as is practiced in Yantra Yoga. Starting in the upper chest, the exhalation moves down to the chest, the lower rib cage, and, lastly, the abdomen. It is the exact reverse of the inhalation, and follows the same vectors of the downward pointing arrowhead-shaped dynamics as the inhalation – but in the opposite direction.

Of course this description of the process of complete exhalation is purely schematic and is meant to give you an idea of the experience.

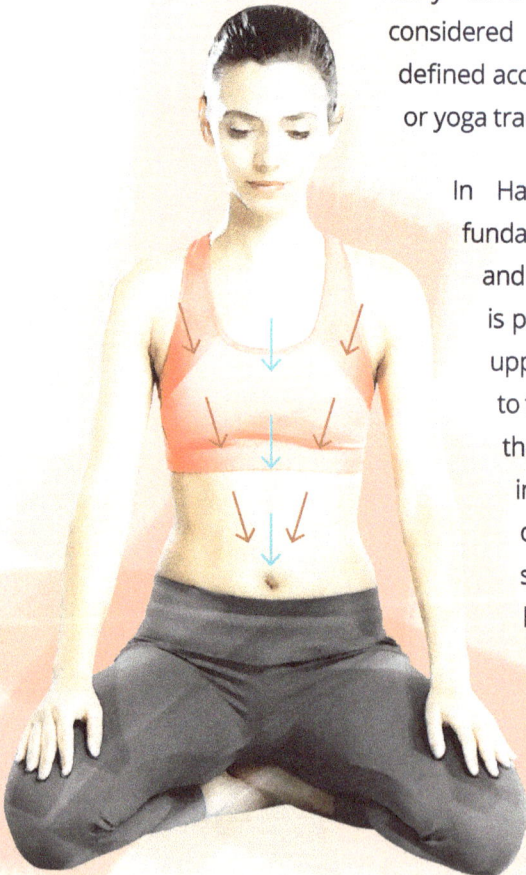

It is not what is really happening. The air is not actually moving out from your chest or your abdomen, but is coming out of the body via the respiratory system.

In this case we are focusing on the inherent elasticity of the lungs, and you can easily train yourself to exhale smoothly and naturally. If you want to exhale deeply, a more active engagement of different muscles is required.

Aim to develop a smooth, direct, unhindered, and continuous flow – without controlling, blocking, or "working" the air in the glottis or back of the throat.

In Harmonious Breathing, we use a four-stage exercise to develop complete exhalation. If you find it comfortable, you can do it sitting on your heels, as shown here, but it is just as effective in a standing position or seated on a chair, as long as you follow the guidelines given earlier for keeping the spine straight and aligned.

Remember to never overdo these kinds of exercises. Do not do them too quickly, too strongly, or for too long.

The experience will be more clear and the effect more precise if you carry out each phase with intent and vigor, alternating with a phase of nonaction.

In response to the effect of these exercises, your habitual breathing patterns will change and come into balance, gradually settling into a different, more natural dynamic.

Although of course inhalation and exhalation are interdependent and the quality of one therefore depends on the other, while practicing each stage of this exercise pay attention mainly to the exhalation phase. The movements will train you to exhale from the chest first, with a gradual closing of the rib cage, and from the abdomen last.

Sometimes it can be useful to introduce a short, relaxed pause after exhalation. This generally allows for a fuller expansion of the breathing and a clearer experience of starting the inhalation from below.

What happens when we pause, especially after an exhalation, is actually just an expansion of our natural physiological pattern of breathing, which spontaneously includes a brief pause after inhalation and a slightly longer one after exhalation.

Some breathwork approaches warn us never to hold the breath. One of the reasons is that doing so might create a tendency to hold the breath after inhaling and after exhaling even in our "everyday" respiration, thus fragmenting the flow of the breathing. Fragmenting the breathing is always considered an erroneous breathing pattern.

In reality, if we train these pauses correctly and gain smooth, gentle, spontaneous control over our respiration, we will achieve exactly the opposite; we will be able to overcome any tendency to block, force, or fragment or unduly tense our breathing. Then, if any circumstances we encounter should influence or restrict our breathing, or if we decide to voluntarily control it, the inner harmony acquired by becoming familiar with softly controlling our inhalations and exhalations will allow us to keep our respiration strong and yet dissolve the tension.

STAGE 1

👍 EASY

The first stage of this set gives you an experiential understanding of the arrowhead shape of inhaling from the bottom up and exhaling from the top down.

Sit on your heels with one foot on top of the other, or next to the other, the knees open, and your hands on your knees.

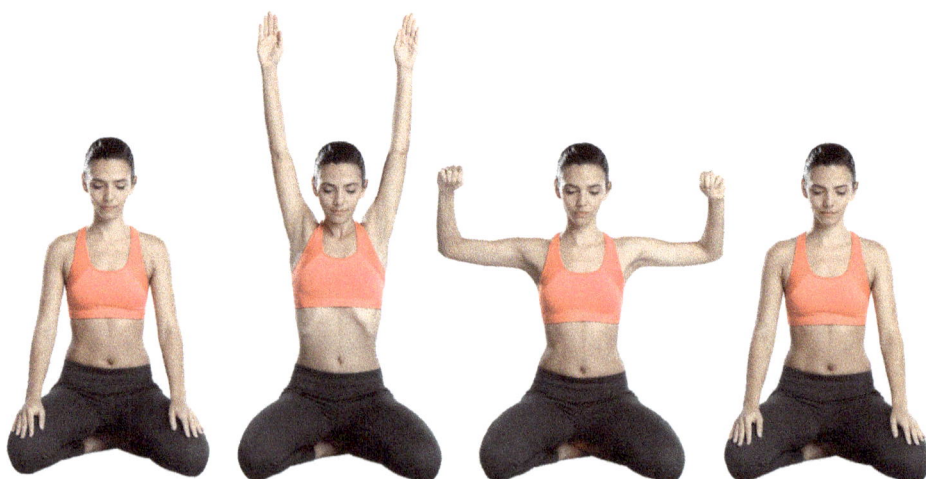

Alternatively, use any of the positions described in the beginning of this part of the book.

Inhale slowly and smoothly from the bottom up, extending the arms up straight above the head and opening them a little to the sides toward the end.

The arm movement trains the upward motion of the air expanding and rising in an ideal pattern, as if along the central shaft of the arrowhead shape.

In a single exhalation, close your hands into fists and lower them as you move the elbows out horizontally at shoulder level and then continue moving them down toward your sides to conclude the exhalation by opening your fists and placing the hands on the knees.

Even though this movement is designed to help you exhale from the upper chest first, then from the chest, the lower rib cage, and lastly the abdomen, it is your presence and your understanding of its purpose that will make the difference, helping you discover a deeper experience and build a more stable capacity.

In a single inhalation starting from below, reach your arms out wide to the sides and slightly back with your palms down and open your chest to the expansion of the air, ending with your arms up alongside the head as you complete the inhalation.

This arm movement trains the upward motion of the air following the direction of the two sides of the arrowhead shape.

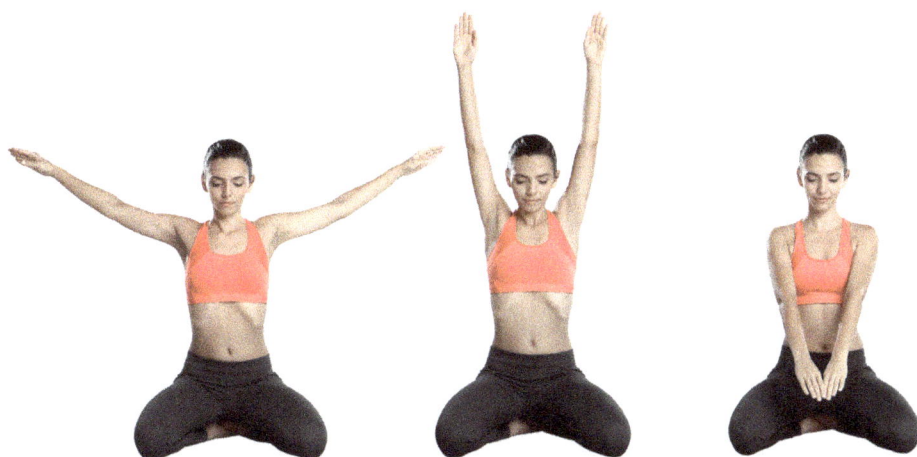

Without blocking or tensing at the top of the inhalation, start to exhale smoothly as you join your hands first and gradually bring the arms down between your knees, emptying the chest first and the abdomen last.

This arm movement trains the downward motion of the air following the direction of the central shaft of the arrowhead shape.

Repeat the entire sequence three to five times; then place your hands on the knees and observe the natural, spontaneous dynamics of the breathing.

Observe whether the exercise has affected the way you breathe, and if so, in what way it has changed.

STAGE 2

 EASY

In the second stage, we change the arm movements slightly to emphasize the experience of exhaling from the chest first.

Sit in the same starting position.

Inhale, raising the arms straight up from the shoulders, and then slightly open them out to the sides.

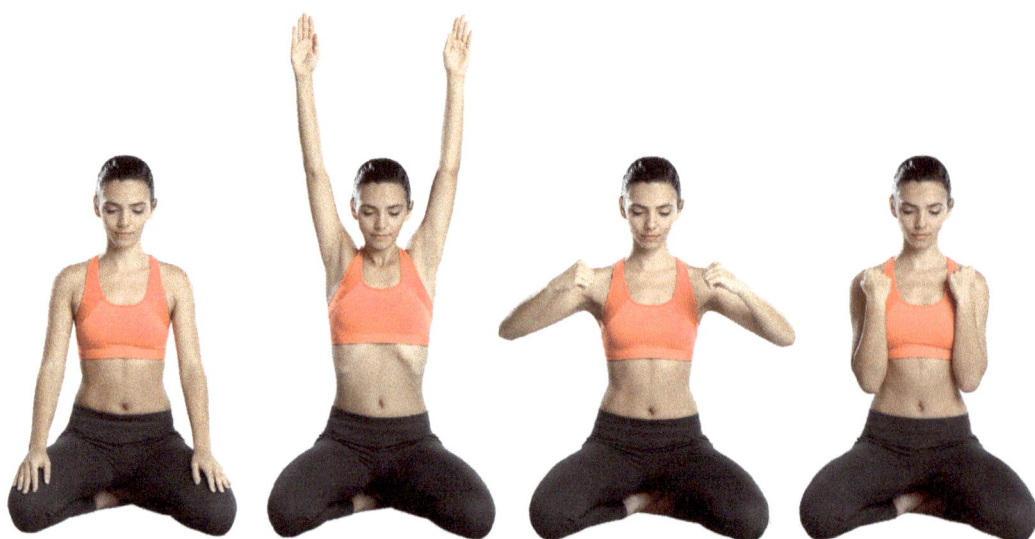

On a single exhalation, make fists and lower them toward the shoulders, with the elbows initially opening out laterally and then closing against your sides as you bring the fists to the front of the shoulders. Keep the back firm throughout this sequence.

The dynamics of the movement help compress the rib cage in such a way as to cause the exhalation to begin in the upper chest and then to move downward, following the action of the movement to end with a contraction of the abdominal muscles.

Inhale, opening the arms out to the sides and then raising them straight overhead.

As in Stage 1, without blocking or tensing at the top of the inhalation, start to exhale smoothly as you join your hands and bring the arms down between your knees. Empty the chest first and the abdomen last.

Repeat no more than three to five times, then place your hands on the knees and relax, breathing and observing.

If you find the position tiring, feel free to change it; move your legs a bit and when you are ready find what feels to be the most comfortable position.

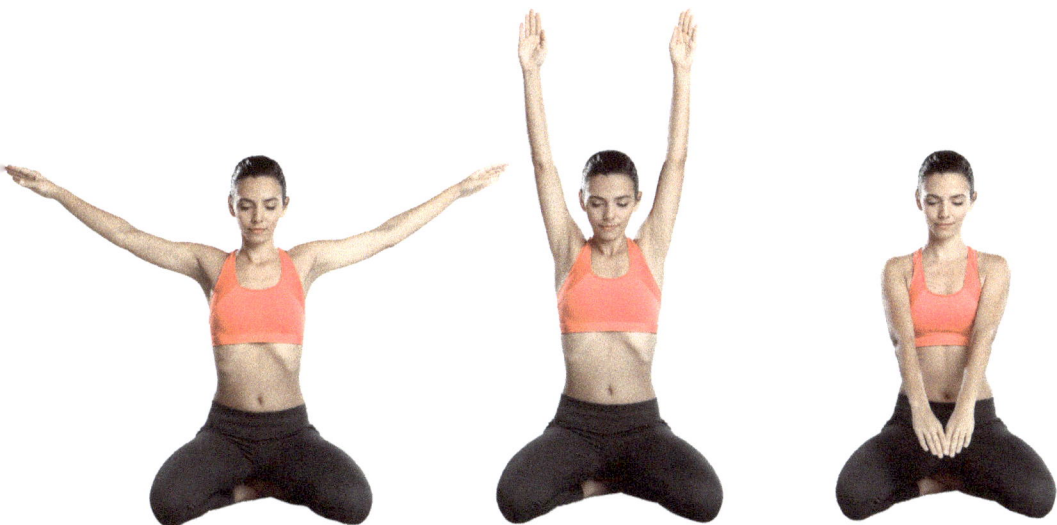

👍 EASY

The third and fourth stages focus more specifically on the upper chest exhalation and at the same time the upper chest expansion.

Sit in the same starting position. Inhale, raising the arms straight up.

On a single exhalation, make fists and lower them toward the shoulders, with the elbows initially opening out laterally and then rotating close to each other in front of your torso as you bring the fists to the front of the shoulders.

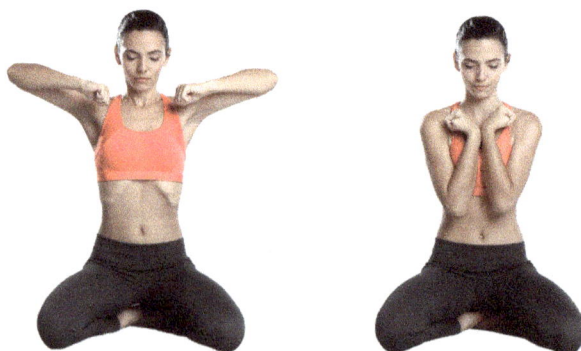

Now inhale, raising the elbows up and out to the sides while continuing to stretch the elbows and fists a bit farther apart and expanding the upper chest even more to help create more space to be filled by the inhalation.

Without blocking in any way, and using the extra stretch to allow for a smooth, fluid exhalation, breathe out as you rotate the forearms to bring the fists in front of the shoulders and the elbows toward each other in front of your torso.

Repeat the entire sequence no more than three times, then rest in the position. Breathe and observe.

STAGE 4

👍 EASY

The fourth stage is done in almost exactly the same way as the third. The only difference is in the central exhalation.

Instead of bringing the fists in front of the shoulders and the elbows tightly closed to the sides, join the elbows and the fists at the center of the chest, thoroughly squeezing the air out of the rib cage and abdomen.

Repeat the entire sequence no more than three times, then place your hands on your knees and rest in the position. Observe the flow of your respiration.

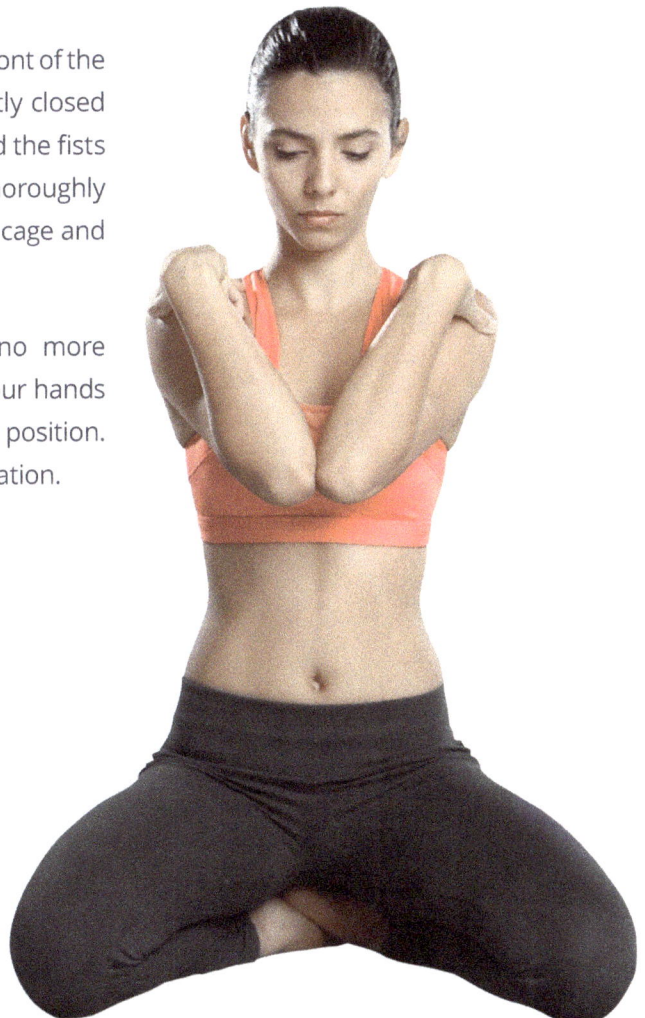

👍 EASY

A slight variation is another useful tool for training the process and dynamics of top-to-bottom exhalation. This same exercise is included in the warm-ups, except that there the coordination of the breath is optional.

Sitting on your heels with the knees comfortably apart, inhale and bring your hands to the top of your shoulders. Exhaling, lower your elbows and then begin to rotate them upward until they meet in front of your chest. Inhaling, open your elbows up and out as you rotate your shoulders back. Exhaling, bring your elbows down in a circular direction and join them in front again.

Repeat this circular motion a few times.

Then inhale as you rotate your elbows in the opposite direction and exhale as you join your elbows at the chest.

Repeat an equal number of times.

Finally, alternate the rotation of the movement, doing one rotation in each direction and coordinating each rotation with the corresponding phase of breathing.

Breathe without forcing, but with intent and energy.

End by placing your hands on the knees and taking a few relaxed breaths. Observe and experience.

RHYTHMIC BREATHING

R hythmic Breathing is an important part of the practice of Yantra Yoga. However, it can benefit anyone, regardless whether they practice yoga. A number of other systems use a similar dynamic in breathing exercises.

In this breathing method we apply a pattern of rhythmic counts to coordinate and improve the individual phases of our breathing.

The uniquely balanced ratio between inhalation, open hold, and exhalation/ empty hold helps us greatly expand our breathing capacity while making it calm and complete, with a continuous, uninterrupted, and natural flow.

It balances our energy and can be a highly effective tool for calming stress and nervousness and resolving mild depression and anxiety.

There is a direct connection between the heartbeat and breathing cycles, and Rhythmic Breathing helps us synchronize the two.

Since our heart rate already naturally increases with each inhalation and decreases with each exhalation, it follows that in particular when the exhalations are longer than the inhalations, our heartbeat can slow down noticeably and have a relaxing effect.

Rhythmic Breathing regulates not only the inhalation and exhalation rates, but also the phase of holding the breath, both after inhalation and after exhalation. This enhances all the qualities and benefits that come from a balanced respiratory rhythm.

The key to this exercise is to maintain presence without distraction, mindfully following the flow of the breath and focusing your attention on the four phases of Rhythmic Breathing: inhalation, open hold, exhalation, and empty hold.

THE PRACTICE

👍 EASY

Sit in any comfortable position with the back straight, shoulders open, and your hands on your knees.

If you are doing Rhythmic Breathing as a stand-alone practice, before you begin, perform the Purification Breathing exercise.

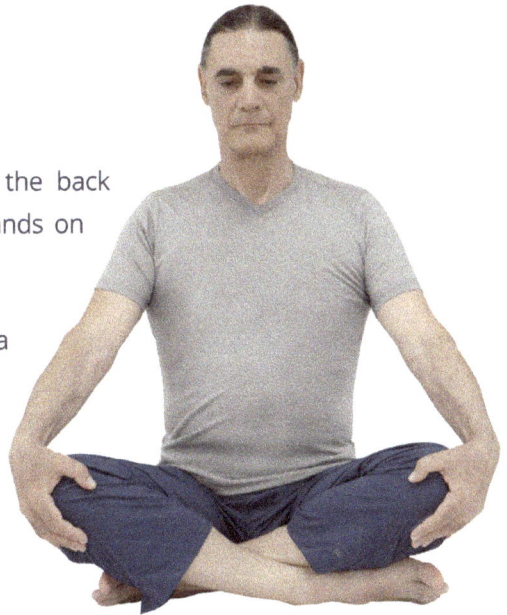

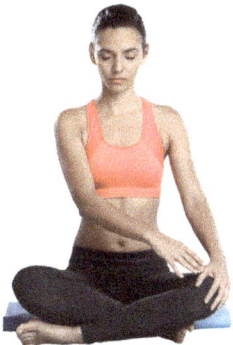

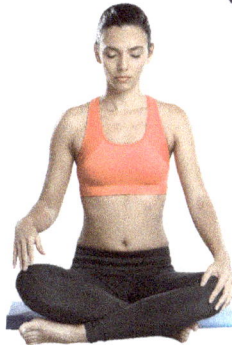

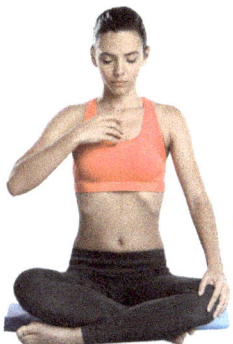

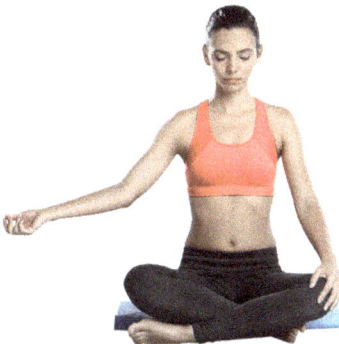

In Rhythmic Breathing we use our right hand to count the rhythm, touching first the left knee, then the right knee, then the center of the chest, and finally clicking the fingers above the right knee. This is the basic count of four.

Using your hand is a simple but effective method to count the rhythm and is easy to learn. In addition, it can help you remain more calm and concentrated.

Alternatively, if it makes it easier for you to keep a constant rhythm, you can use a metronome. If you find the hand motion distracting, it is also possible to just count in your mind, without moving your hand. Simply remain relaxed but present in your sitting position and breathe according to the rhythm.

The rhythm starts at four counts, each count ideally corresponding to, or at least not faster than, the heartbeat of a healthy person in a relaxed state.

Of course the pace depends on our individual condition and capacity, but it is good to try to keep it on the slow side – without forcefully pushing past our limits. Instead, we just try to gently overcome our limitations.

When we apply a count of six – or any multiple of four plus two – we count four normally and for the last two counts, touch the center of the chest once again and then again click the fingers above the right knee to complete the sixth count.

BREATHING METHOD

In the first round, start with four counts for the inhalation, four counts for the open retention, and four counts for the exhalation. The exhalation is divided into two counts of actual exhalation and two of empty retention. The empty hold in the second part of the exhalation process can be experienced as a kind of passive continuation of the actual exhalation.

Make sure that the inhalation is complete, beginning in the abdomen and expanding out to the sides and up to the chest in a direct, relaxed, smooth, and calm flow through the nostrils.

Now hold for four counts, keeping your hold relaxed and open in your chest. Let it be a relaxed, extended pause in the flow of the breathing, without any tension, blockage, or obstruction.

Then exhale smoothly in two counts, initially increasing the strength and flow of the air, then decreasing it gradually and entering into a relaxed and tension-free empty hold for two counts.

There is no specified number of repetitions for this breathing exercise; you can repeat it as many times as is suitable for you.

If at any time you feel any difficulty or tension, or each time you change the count, apply one or three deep exhalations as in the Purification Breathing exercise.

With training you can progress from 4-4-4 to the next count of the rhythm: 4-6-4, inhaling four counts, holding six counts, and exhaling four counts (of which two counts are active exhalation and two empty retention).

The next rhythm is 4-6-6, inhaling four counts, holding six counts, and exhaling six counts (of which three counts are active exhalation and three empty retention).

The last rhythm we generally use in Harmonious Breathing is 4-6-8. This rhythm configuration is generally experienced as comfortable and really helps you develop the capacity and quality of your breathing patterns.

As in Purification Breathing, if possible let the shape of your inhalations be like a grain of barley, opening gradually to an expansion and then gently tapering off at the end. Similarly, let the exhalations start off gradually, broaden in the middle, and then taper off again.

You can use the same counting technique to train only the phases of inhalation and exhalation, without the central hold. It will still be a wonderful breathing exercise, and a good way to calm your mind by gradually increasing the length of the exhalation. In this case, use a count of 4-4, 4-6, and 4-8.

UNIFYING THE FLOW

The next exercise is a particularly enjoyable way to learn how to relax and expand the flow of our breath, dispel tensions, and develop a breathing pattern that is completely free, flexible, and aware.

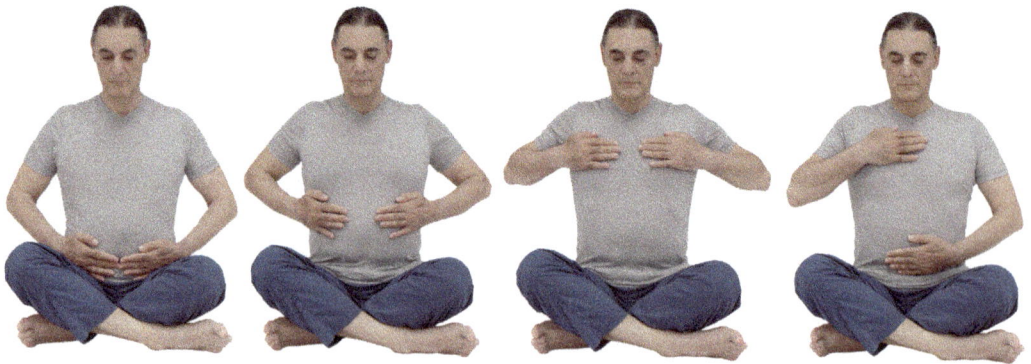

Bring your hands to the abdomen and feel the smooth expansion of the breathing. Do not force anything; let the experience be spontaneous, open, and relaxed.

Then move your hands to the ribs and do the same as before. Feel the expansion focused under your lower rib cage.

Now move your hands to the chest, sensing the expansion and opening.

Finally, put one hand on the abdomen and one on the chest.

Breathe completely and in a relaxed manner, inhaling from the bottom up, and exhaling from the top down. When you inhale, feel the expansion under both hands, first in the abdomen then up in the chest. Expand fully, but without forcing. When you exhale, feel the air moving out from the chest first and concluding in the abdomen in a smooth progression. Let the exhalation be long and deep, softly engaging your abdominal muscles. Let the body breathe, only gently helping the expansion and contraction of the breathing.

You can also practice with similar rhythms as in Rhythmic Breathing, simply applying a brief pause at the top of the inhalation and another brief one at the bottom of the exhalation. Gradually you can increase the pause after inhalation, providing you feel no block or tension.

Another alternative is to inhale, then hold open for a moment, keeping the chest expanded. Then, still holding open, let the chest "settle down." Relax in that inner movement before starting to exhale smoothly and fluidly. This is a highly effective way to train how to transition smoothly from inhalation to exhalation.

You can practice in any position, as long as you keep the back straight and are comfortable, yet alert, with presence, with intent.

POSSIBLE ALTERNATE POSITIONS

Seated on a chair (with or without props)

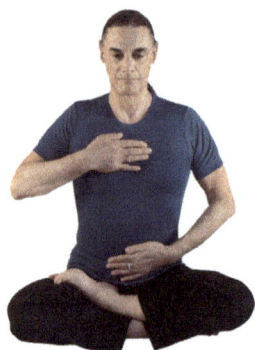

Half lotus

Knees apart

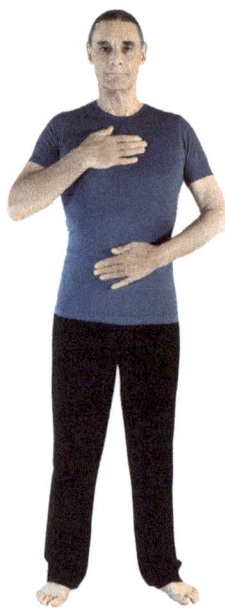

Standing

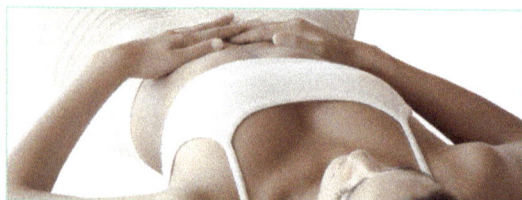

Lying on the floor

With or without props

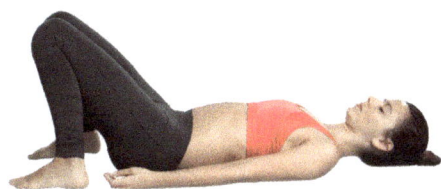

Knees together, feet pointing inward

Knees open, feet pointing outward to the sides

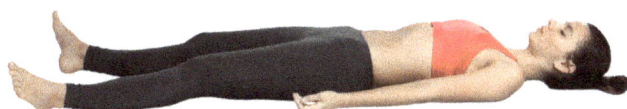

Legs stretched out, feet loosely falling to the sides

In a reclining position, the expansion of the breathing is a little less free with the exception of the abdominal phase, but it is still quite clear and effective, and, especially with the help of some support, the position is very comfortable and ensures a good alignment of the spine.

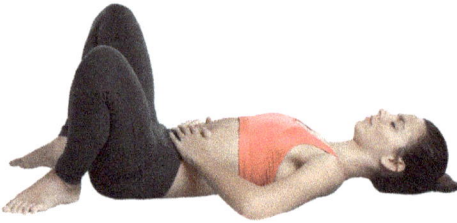

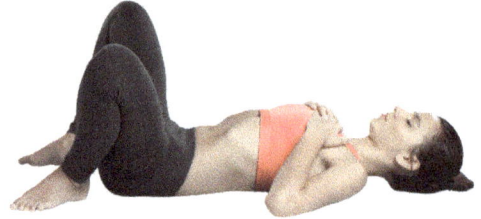

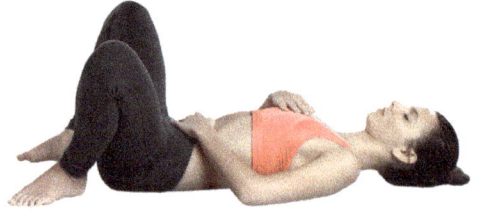

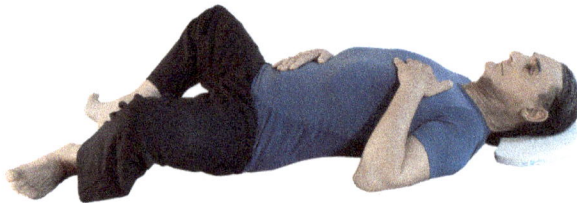

Hand placement for breath observation

NATURAL BREATHING

👍 EASY

This next exercise focuses on making the breathing more flexible and, ultimately, more spontaneous and natural.

Any comfortable position

This exercise can be done in any comfortable sitting position with the back straight as shown before.

Nevertheless, it is quite comfortable – and also most effective – to perform it lying down on the floor with the knees open, heels in front of the buttocks, and feet pointing outward to the sides.

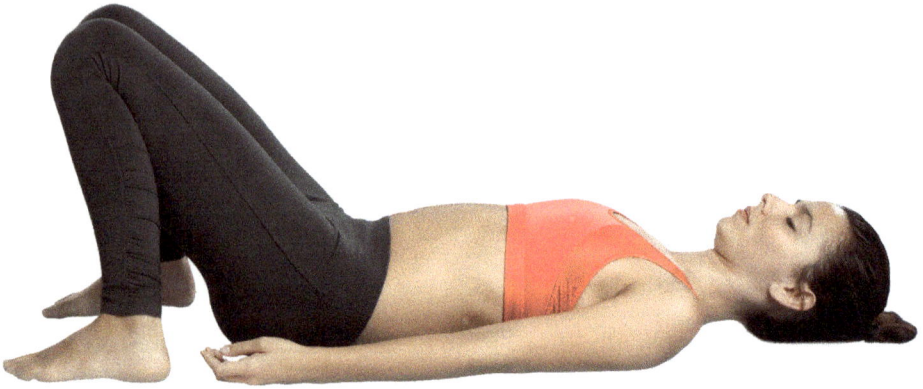

As an alternative, or if you are tired, join your knees, keeping the heels in the same place.

You can keep the arms along the sides or put one hand on the abdomen and the other on the chest to guide your presence.

Natural is a wonderful word that can evoke something pure and beautiful. Something not directly connected to the action of the mind, to judgment and analysis. Something that happens spontaneously and is perfect and harmonious. In reality this can happen only when we are not conditioned by tensions of the mind, energy, and body. As long as we are conditioned by these tensions we cannot fully experience something really natural, something free and pure.

Nevertheless, with training we can get closer to that natural experience. We can "see" how this condition can be, we can see beyond our tensions. We can relax, even if only briefly, in a natural flow of the breathing. With training we can also learn how to connect this smooth flow of the breathing with movements that can even be energetic and powerful without losing their inner grace. We can experience how relaxed breathing in a relaxed body can help relax the mind, relax the tension, the stress. Now we can say we are experiencing a more natural relaxed condition.

If you want to be especially comfortable you can put a pillow under each knee and a support under the head. In this way you will feel absolutely no strain and be able to hold the position even for a long time.

The following description is just an example of how you can do this exercise. You can do it for as long as you like, extending or shortening the individual phases as you please and repeating each as many times as you like, depending how much time you have. Do what feels best for you.

At first, just relax and breathe, naturally, easily, and calmly. Let the breath flow the way it happens spontaneously.

Then start to give a shape to the breathing, try to start in the abdomen and gently move up to the chest.

Breathe gently and evenly, staying within the middle range of your respiration capacity. This is what we call the tidal volume, the volume of air breathed in or out during normal, resting, uncontrolled respiration (see glossary).

After a few breathing cycles start to expand more, keeping the inhalation and the exhalation at the same length and intensity, expanding gradually at the same rate. In technical language, you are now entering your reserve inhalation and reserve exhalation volumes, the range beyond your average capacity. Try to open your inhalation more, but without tensing or blocking.

Let the inhalations smoothly and effortlessly flow into the exhalations, and exhalations into the inhalations.

The exhalations start in the chest and end in the abdomen.

Now start shortening the breathing cycle; keep a constant proportion and rhythm of the respiration but make it shorter and shorter – without compromising the complete, bottom-up dynamics of the breathing.

Then start expanding again as before.

Do each of these phases at least three, five, or seven times.

You can also count the rhythm of your inhalations and exhalations, breathing in for two counts and exhaling for two counts, then three and three, four and four, five and five, if possible going to six counts of inhaling and exhaling.

Then concentrate more on the exhalation, making it longer than the inhalation. Expand well when you inhale, then exhale long and deep.

As with the equal inhalations and exhalations, you can count the rhythm if it helps you keep track: inhale for two counts, exhale for three; inhale for three counts, exhale for four; inhale for four counts, exhale for six. Finally, if possible, inhale for five counts and exhale for eight.

Then again make the inhalations and exhalations the same length and intensity, expanding and exhaling smoothly and without forcing.

In the next phase you can hold a little after inhaling: instead of exhaling immediately, take a brief pause in the breathing – without any tension, without closing, without blocking. Keep a sense of inner expansion.

Smoothly and gracefully exhale, gradually and completely, longer than the inhalation. After exhaling, pause, without immediately inhaling, and relax into the empty space at the bottom of exhalation a little longer than the pause after inhalation.

When you are ready, inhale again and exhale smoothly and fully, this time without pauses.

Continue inhaling and exhaling, gradually making the count of your inhalations and exhalations equal again.

Now concentrate on longer exhalations and on staying empty for a longer time at the bottom of the exhalation. Relax in the empty space and passively wait for the body to open to the spontaneous impulse to inhale. When that happens, take the momentum of the opening inhalation and let it expand fully from the abdomen up to the chest. Then exhale, wait in a relaxed state, and inhale once again.

Repeat a few times, expanding with the inhalation and relaxing with the exhalation.

Now stop pausing at the bottom of the exhalation and let the breath become increasingly passive.

Anytime you feel tired you can change the position of the legs.

Gradually stop deciding how to breathe. Let your body take over, just observe and relax, let the breathing become uncontrolled, soft; let it be spontaneous and free.

Always be mindful of your respiration; whether you are shaping it or letting it be, just be aware of it.

When you want to finish the session stretch your legs out in front, keeping them slightly apart.

Now you are ready to completely relax.

COMPLETE RELAXATION

👍 EASY

To conclude our breathing practice, we simply lie down and relax the tensions we have in our body, let our breath flow spontaneously, naturally, and calmly, and let go of the mind.

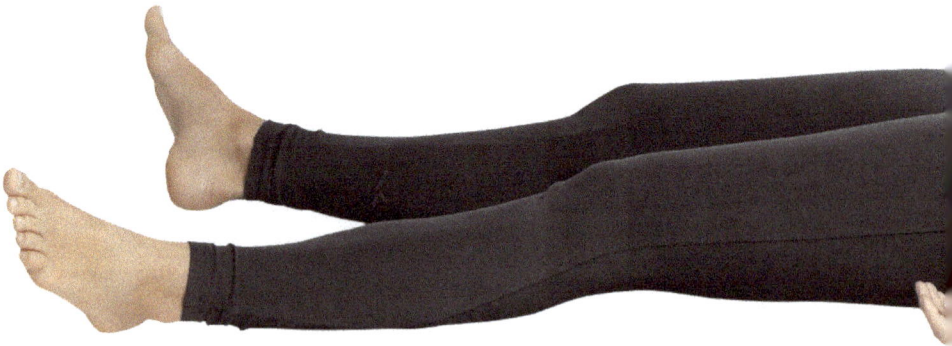

Lying on your back, with your arms loosely to the sides and legs slightly open, just let everything be, without changing or modifying anything. Feel the entire body completely relaxed.

Feel the heaviness of your whole body bearing on the ground, but at the same time remain without any tension, in a vast, open, and free space.

You can also relax gradually, concentrating first on the head, then the arms, the torso, the waist, the legs and feet. Take all the time you need, all the time you like.

Now concentrate on the breathing, let the breathing be free and relaxed; just observe, don't change anything. Let the movement of the breathing be unconditioned.

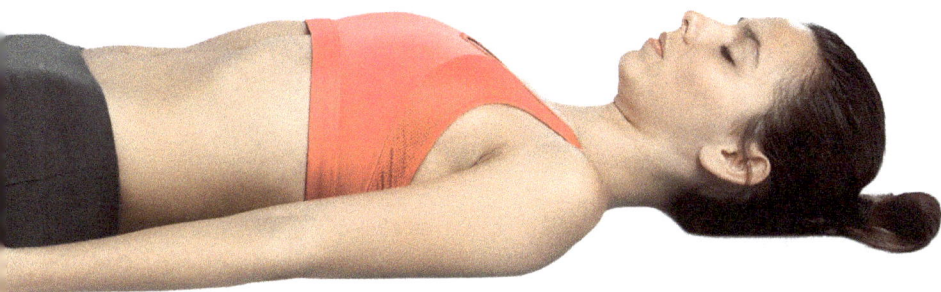

If you feel any tension at all in the breathing, just be aware of it and dissolve it in vast, empty space.

Don't change anything in the mind, don't block or follow the movement of the mind. Just let your mind be free and relaxed.

Let the body, energy, and mind be free, without correcting anything, leaving everything in a naturally relaxed condition.

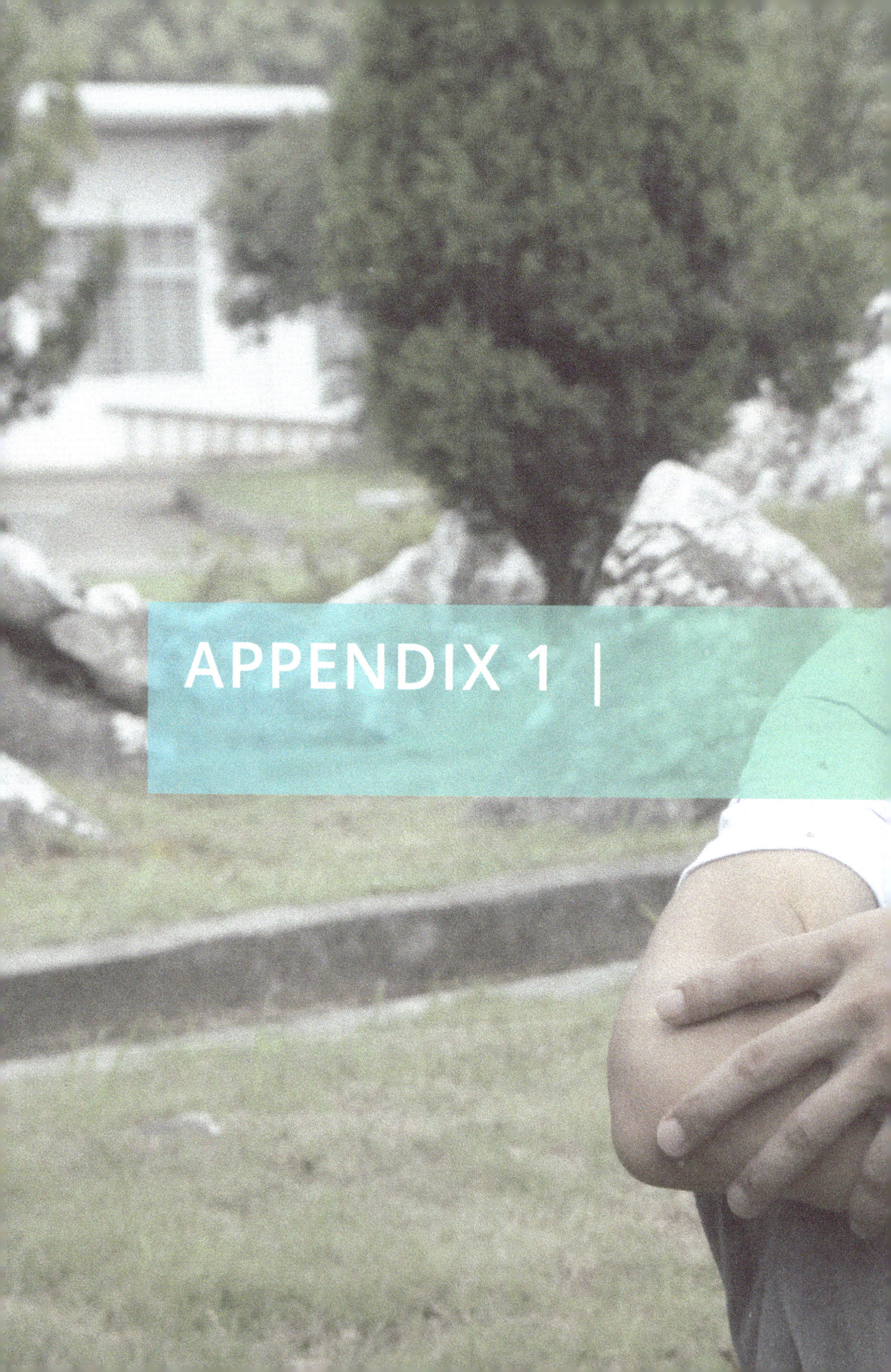

APPENDIX 1 |

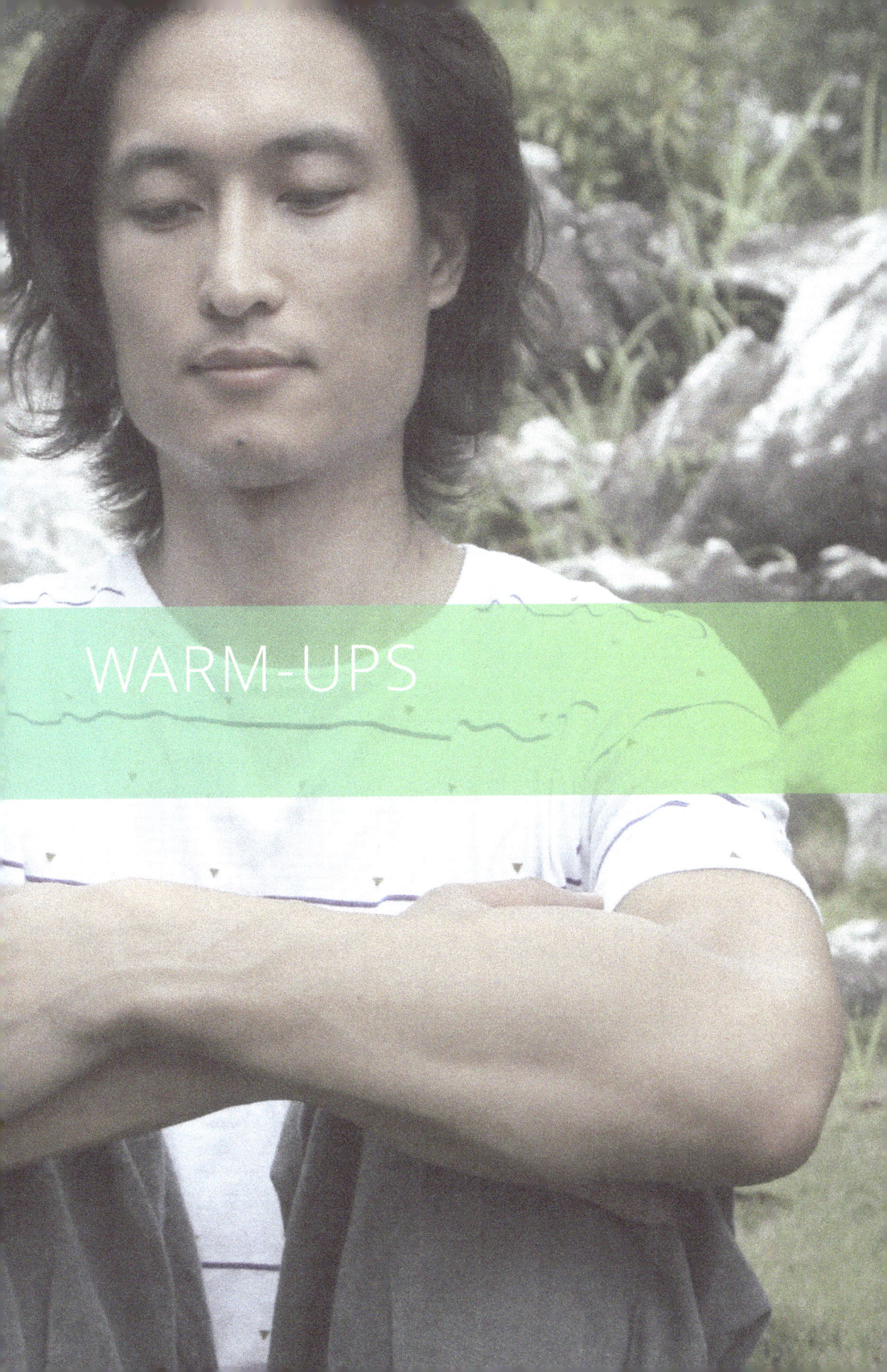

WARM-UPS

WARM-UPS

To get the most out of Harmonious Breathing, it is best to start with some simple warm-ups to help you release tensions and prepare your body. This section on warm-ups is included as an appendix because although these exercises can improve the quality of your breathwork, they are an adjunct rather than the core practice. The selection presented here will help you apply the exercises to open up your breathing more correctly and without effort or tension. They will also contribute to developing an the optimum posture for seated breathing exercises. More generally, these warm-ups encourage the best possible alignment of the spine, which plays such a vital role in taking care of our body. Each of these simple exercises also has specific benefits, such as tonifying the related muscles or loosening the activated joints.

If you have the desire and the time, you can practice the entire series of warm-ups, or just the ones you find most useful and easiest.

As with any exercises, never force or strain. Let the movements – as well as the breathing – be smooth and harmonious. Always listen to the body, energy, and mind, and work with your particular circumstances.

In general, these exercises can be repeated three to five times each, but there is no fixed rule or routine. For the most part, you can do them as many times as you like, depending on the amount of time you have and what feels right at the moment. You can also do them in any order that suits you. A basic guideline is to begin with easier exercises, and alternate the ones that are active with those that are more static.

In the more active exercises, the breathing is coordinated with the movements; the static ones emphasize relaxing in the main position and breathing naturally and fluidly without forcing any structure on the breathing.

GENERAL POINTERS ON BREATHING

Keeping your experience fresh, simple, and clear will release the full potential of stress-free breathing. So it is important never to overdo the training and instead to take pauses, observe, and discover.

In the beginning it is better not to impose a specific structure on the breathing. As much as possible, keep the respiration fluid and without fragmentation or tension. At first, keep within what is called the tidal volume of the respiration – your normal range – then slowly you can start to expand the range more actively.

For every movement we perform, and in every position we pause, in one way or another the breathing is always influenced and shaped by that position or movement.

As an example, a physical position that involves a closing of the chest will impair full chest breathing. A position that expands the chest, on the other hand, will favor full chest breathing.

Movements and positions change the shape of the body and consequently also influence the breathing.

More interestingly, but less evident, is that the way we breathe influences not only our position, but also the way we move and the dynamics of the movement.

This interdependence between position, movement, and breathing is what makes it possible to train, or retrain, our breathing to be complete, fluid, and harmonious. This is a truth you can experience in everyday life.

If you are agitated your respiration will be constricted and agitated. Conversely, if you are calm and emotionally tension-free, your breathing will be calmer and smoother.

If you coordinate your breathing, you will coordinate your energy and relax your mind.

You will experience a more aware, calm, clear, and vital mind and a new energy in your life. You will also develop a healthier body.

CREATING A WARM-UP ROUTINE

Even though the warm-ups presented here follow a particular structure to guide you and help you understand the principle of what you are doing and why, ultimately they are suggestions only. You have to make them your own. Only you know your body, breathing, and mind. Only you can really experience the totality of your condition and discover what it is best for you. You are the best trainer you can have.

Just try to be aware and present, not distracted. Be present in what you do. Just observe and discover.

Often, common sense works better than any set of complicated instructions. If done with attention and without tension, often the simpler the exercise, the better. More advanced exercises may naturally bring a fuller sense of accomplishment, but when done correctly it is the simple exercises that can provide a particularly clear and useful experience. If performed with this understanding, simplicity is powerful.

As with the core exercises presented in part 2, we can divide the warm-up exercises roughly into three categories:

1. 👍 EASY

2. 👉 MODERATE

3. 👎 CHALLENGING

However, none of these warm-up exercises are really difficult to perform.

The exercises selected here address six main actions to warm up and train the overall flexibility and tone of the body, and especially the spine:

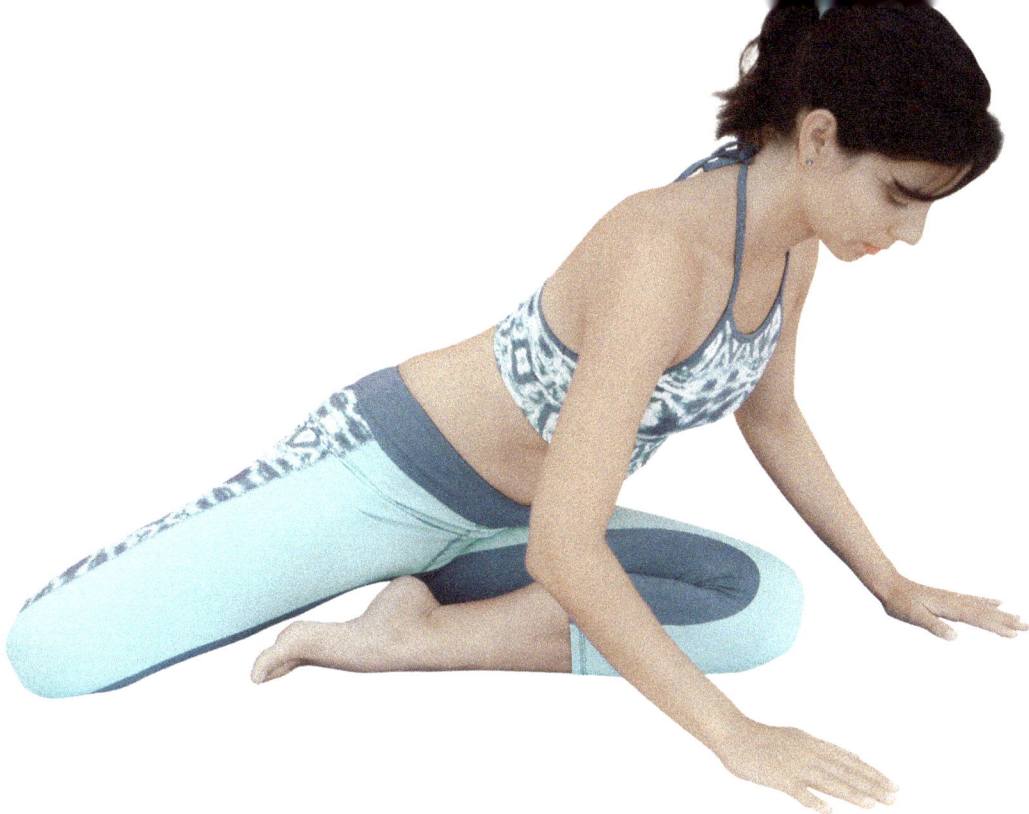

1. Bending forward

2. Arching backward

3. Stretching the left side

4. Stretching the right side

5. Twisting to the left

6. Twisting to the right

It is generally advisable to start a session of warm-ups with one or more of the dynamic standing exercises. Alternatively you can start with the neck and shoulder exercises at the end of this section. If possible, in each session perform at least one exercise for each of the above categories.

Then, if you have decided to concentrate on a particular series of breathing exercises during your practice session, you can focus on warm-ups that will make those movements easier to perform and more precise. Choose the warm-ups that are most effective for you. Whenever possible, coordinate your breathing with the movements. Let your inhalations and exhalations be relaxed, but filled with a sense of vigor, presence, and energy. In almost all of the warm-ups, the quality of the breathing should be complete, calm, and smooth. In general we inhale when the position is expanding and opening and exhale when position is closing or contracting.

STANDING WARM-UPS

SWINGING

👍 EASY

Training Focus: Gently mobilizes the lower back, loosens the arms and shoulders, and helps synchronize movement and breathing.

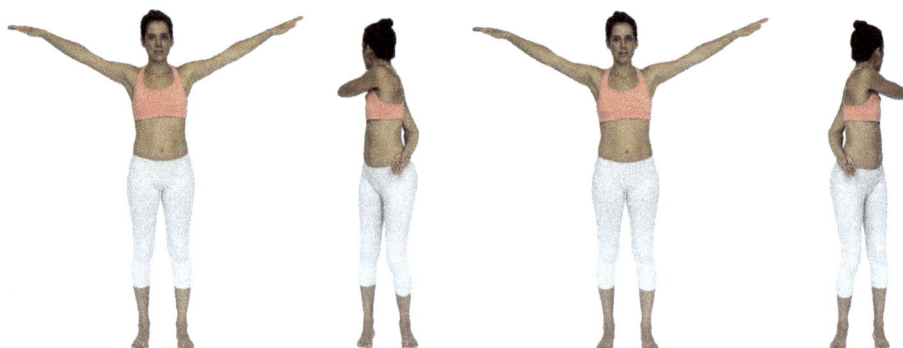

Stand relaxed yet present, with your feet at least a shoulder width apart.

Inhaling, open your arms out wide.

Exhaling, swing your arms around your hips, turning to one side and rotating your spine.

Inhaling, come back to the center while opening your arms out wide.

Then exhale, turning to the other side, wrapping your arms around your hips. Repeat three to five times or as many times as feels right to you at this moment.

BENDING FORWARD

👍 MODERATE

Training Focus: Relaxes and lengthens the spine, releases tension.

Stand with your arms along the sides. Be sure that even when standing, you are present, comfortable, and gently controlled with the best possible alignment. Breathe calmly.

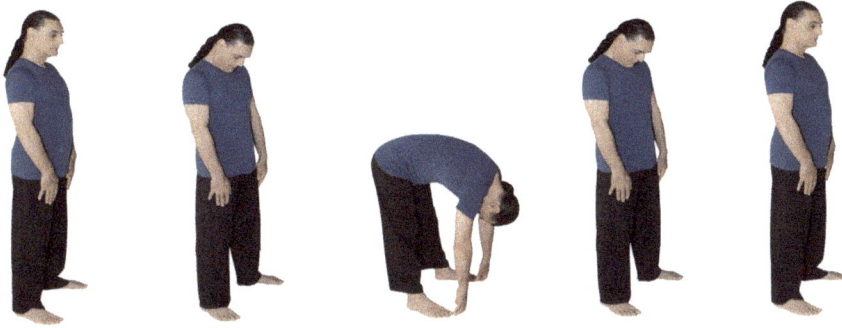

Exhaling, gradually bend forward. First, drop your chin toward the chest. Then, keeping your waist and legs controlled, let the weight of gravity bear on your arms and head, drawing them toward the floor. Relax and let the arms and head passively hang.

If you cannot manage to reach down in a single exhalation, you can stop midway and inhale smoothly. Then exhale once more, continuing to move the arms and head toward the ground. If you find this too challenging, especially on the lower back, you can bend your knees a little to release any tension. This two-step approach can be thought of as a preparation – a warm-up for a warm-up, as it were. What you are working toward is to be able to bend all the way down with a single, complete exhalation and straighten all the way back up with a single, coordinated inhalation.

When you reach the farthest you can comfortably bend forward, stay there and rest a little, breathing gently. You can also remain for a moment in empty hold before coming up as you inhale.

Then inhale as you gradually straighten your torso, keeping the legs rooted and the waist firmly in place. Keep the head looking down until your whole torso is upright, and only then raise the chin to straighten the head.

Take a couple of gentle breath cycles in standing position and then start again.

You can repeat the exercise a few times. It is a wonderful practice in the morning, done according to your capacity. It will tune you up for the beginning of a new day.

ARM CIRCLES

👍 MODERATE

Training Focus: Shoulder joints.

Stand and open your arms, firmly engaged, out to the sides. Inhaling and exhaling normally, make small circles with the arms, rotating from the shoulder joints, first in one direction, then in the other.

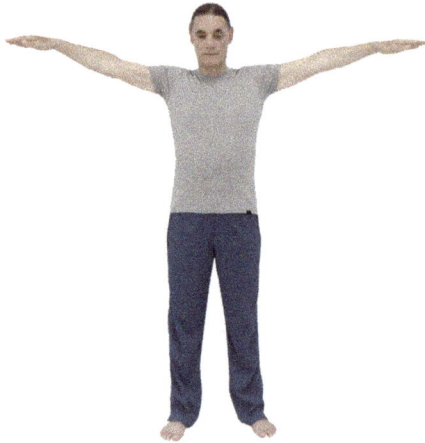

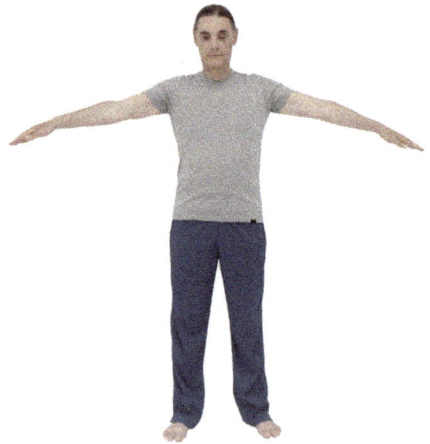

THE TREE

👍 MODERATE

Training Focus: All movements involving balance are helpful in calming the mind and making us more aware of our breathing.

Stand relaxed yet present, with your feet slightly apart and parallel, arms along your sides. Use your hand to bring the sole of one foot to the top of the inner thigh of your other leg.

Breathe calmly and balance on your standing leg.

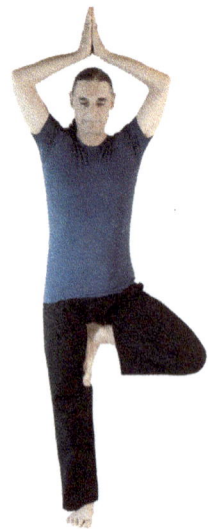

Slowly raise your arms to join your hands above your head, standing on one leg as long as the pose is comfortable and easy.

To help you maintain your balance, focus on an unmoving spot in the distance or something static in front of you on the floor.

Then slowly bring your hands back down while lowering your foot to the floor, returning to the starting position with your arms along your sides.

Repeat the exercise on the other side.

KNEE STRENGTHENER

 MODERATE

Training Focus: Increases strength and flexibility of the hips, knees, and ankles.

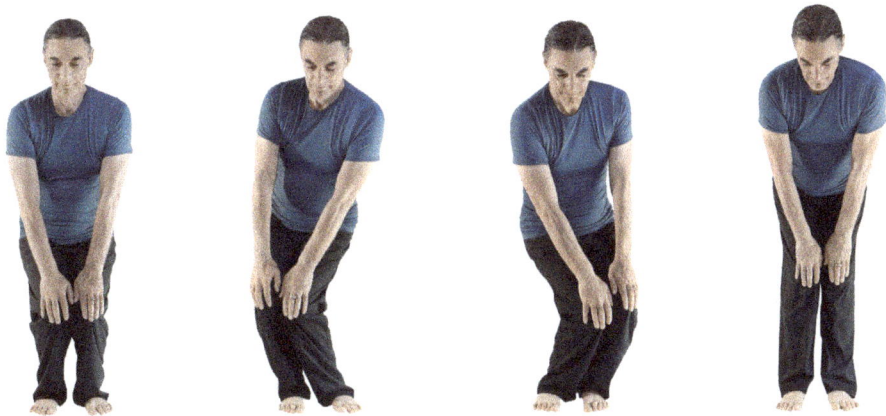

From standing, bend your knees and put your hands on them. Inhaling and exhaling normally, rotate the knees in one direction a few times, bending and straightening the legs to facilitate the movement. Then rotate in the other direction.

SQUAT

👆CHALLENGING

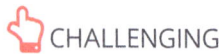

Training Focus: Increases strength of the knees and legs, lengthens the spine, and increases flexibility of the hips and ankles.

This exercise is very effective, but can be quite challenging for the knees, so if you have any knee problems, or feel it is too demanding or difficult, it is better not to perform it.

Stand relaxed yet present, with your feet slightly apart and parallel or the toes pointing slightly outward, arms along your sides. Inhale, raising your arms parallel in front to shoulder level. Exhale as you bend your knees and squat down toward your heels, going only as far as is comfortable and keeping your feet as flat on the floor as possible. Inhale, rising back up and keeping your arms in front. Repeat three to five times.

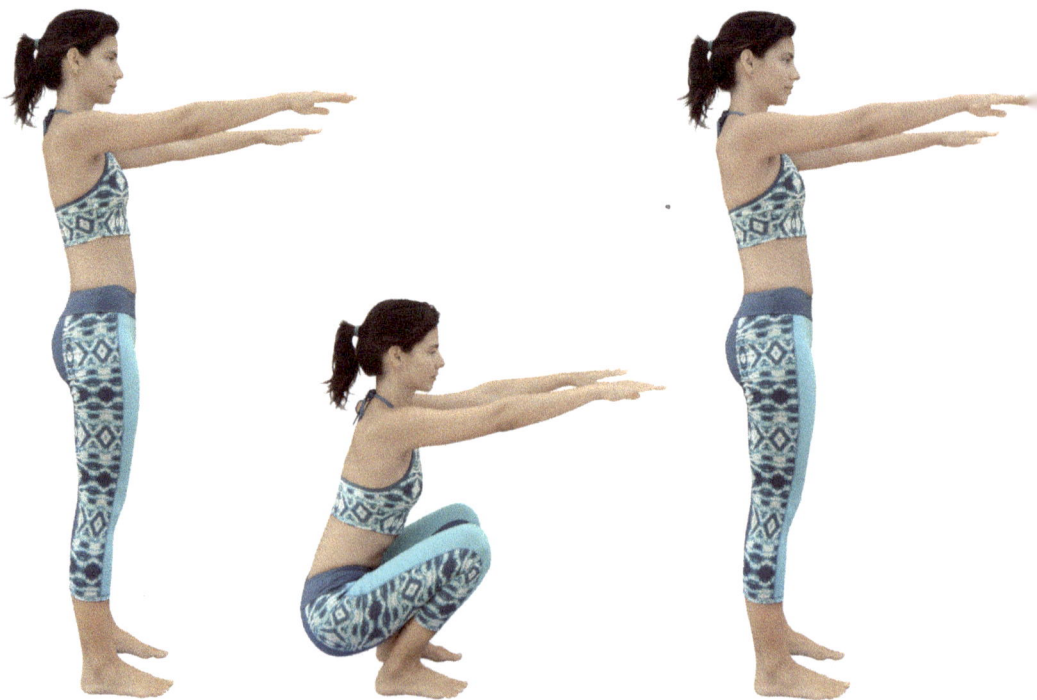

This exercise can also be done with a small mat or a blanket under your heels to make it easier and help you develop a deeper squat.

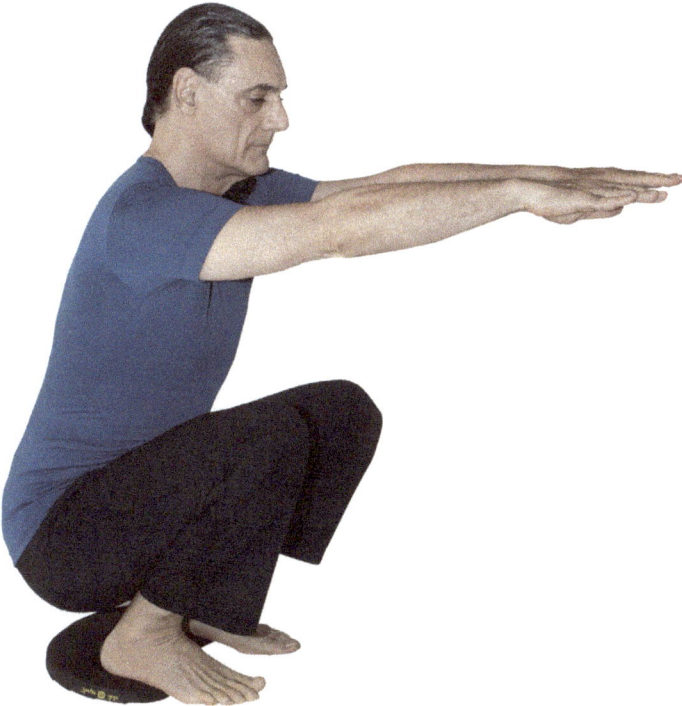

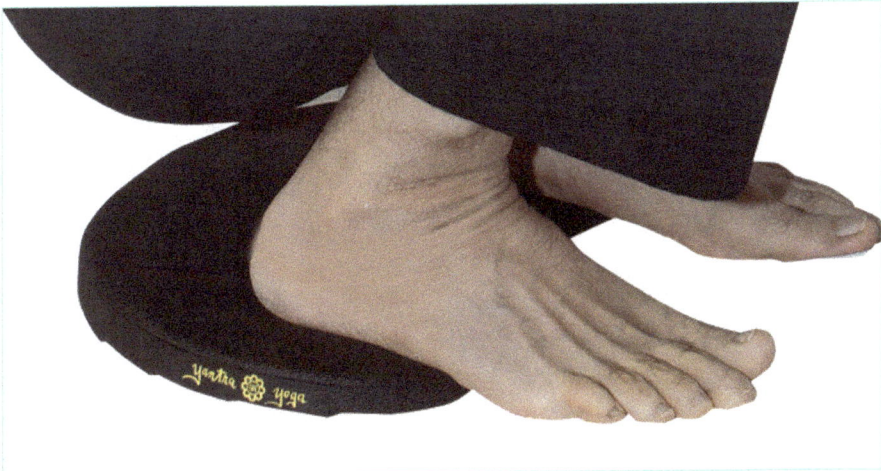

SEATED WARM-UPS

ROTATE AND FLEX HANDS AND FEET

👍 EASY

Training Focus: Keeps hands and feet flexible and pain free while also stretching the muscles of the limbs.

A good way to start the day is to move hands and feet in this way while still in bed, just after you wake up.

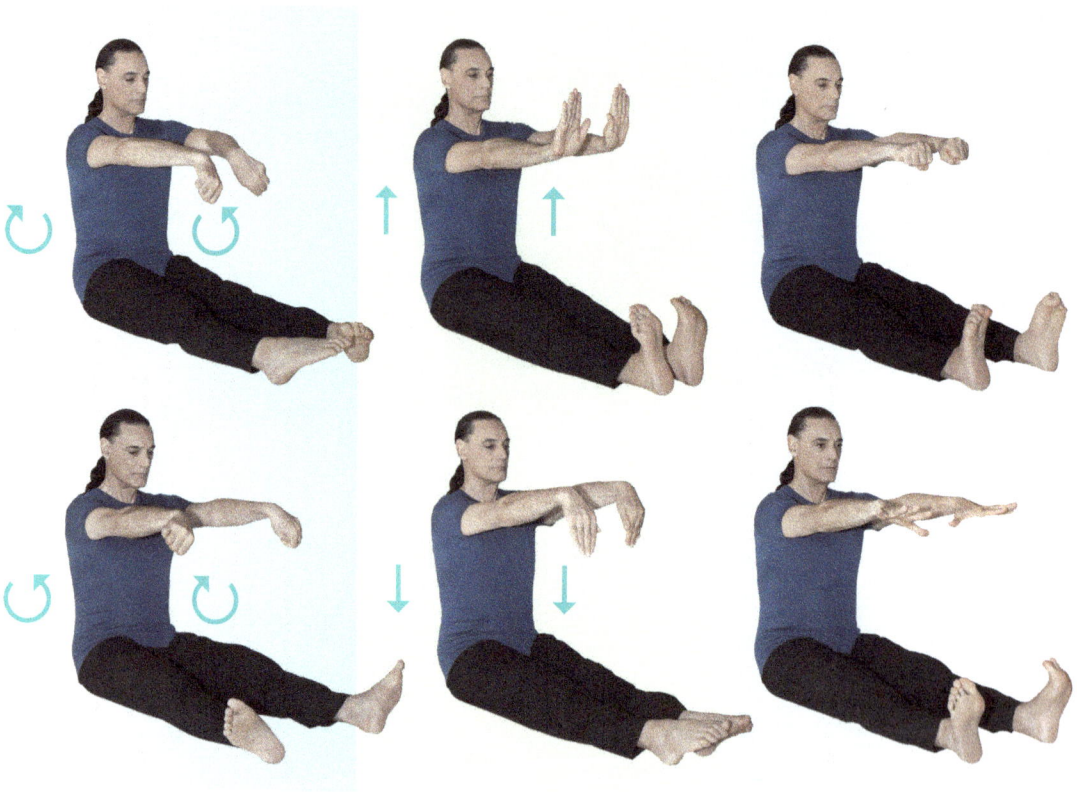

Sit with your legs and arms straight out in front and parallel. Inhale and exhale normally as you rotate your hands and feet simultaneously, first in one direction and then in the other. Then, flex and point your feet and also flex your hands both up and down, following the direction of your feet. Finally, curl your toes and open them apart while closing your hands in a fist and then spreading the fingers out wide as you move your hands and feet and breathe normally.

If in the beginning you find it difficult to coordinate the movement of the feet and hands, you can train each part separately, rotating the hands first and then the feet.

SHAKING THE FEET

👍 EASY

Training Focus: Mobilizes and eliminates excess fluid from the toes and feet and improves the flexibility of the ankles.

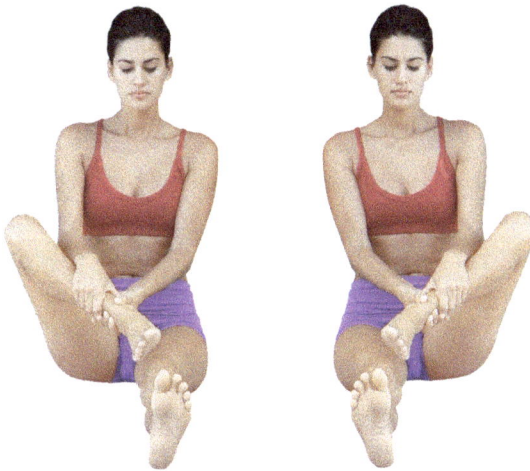

Sitting on the floor with your back straight and your legs out parallel in front, take hold of one foot by the ankle with both hands, bring it in front of your torso, and shake it vigorously. After a while, stop shaking it and stretch the leg in out front, then take hold of the other ankle and shake the other foot. Continue to alternate three to five times.

As you inhale and exhale through the nose, the breathing should be continuous and relaxed.

You can also take hold of both ankles and shake them vigorously while balancing on your buttocks.

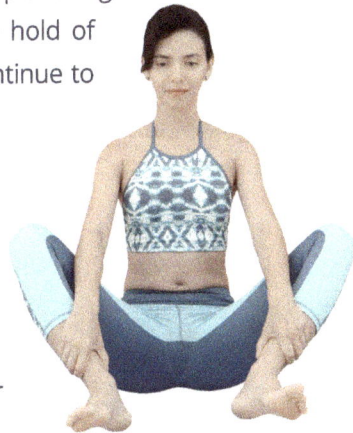

SWINGING THE LOWER LEGS

👍 EASY

Training Focus: Mobilizes knees and ankles, eliminates excess fluid from the joints of the knees and feet.

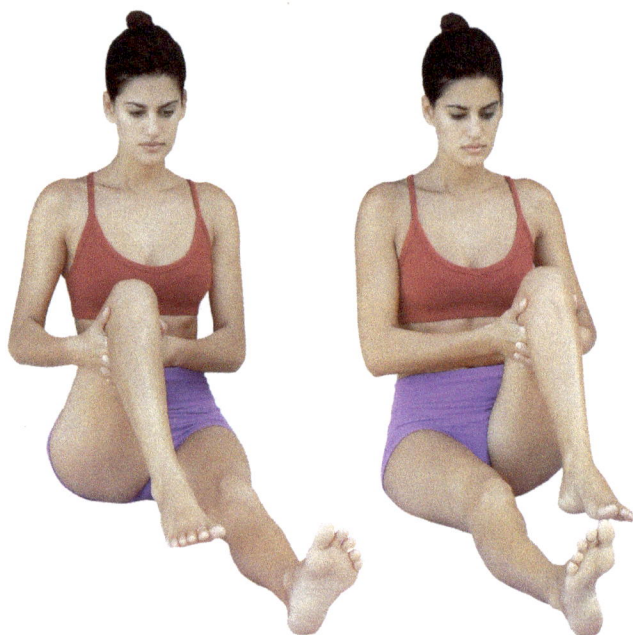

Sit on the floor with one leg stretched out in front and one leg bent so that your foot is beside the other knee. Take hold of your bent leg above the knee joint with both hands, interlacing your fingers and placing the thumbs on each side of the knee. Move the knee from side to side, allowing the lower leg to swing freely, three to five times, keeping the leg and knee joint loose and relaxed. Keep the abdominal muscles firm to stabilize the body.

Repeat with the other leg, alternating a few times.

KNEE TO THE SIDE

👍 MODERATE

Training Focus: Mobilizes the knee joints.

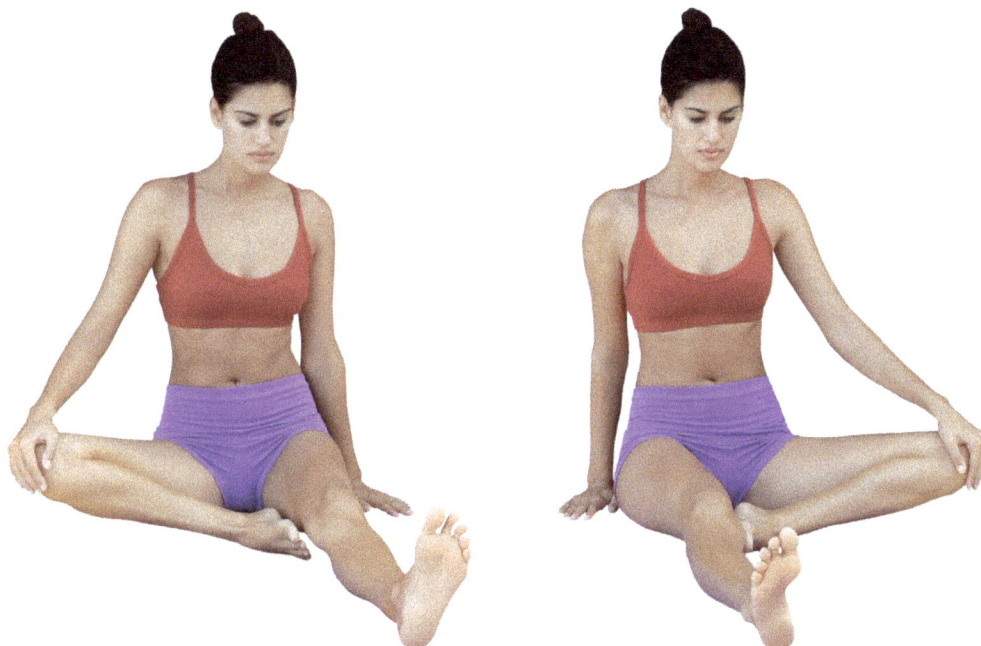

Sitting with your legs straight out in front and a hand on each knee, inhale smoothly.

Exhale as you bend one knee outward, bring the foot toward the perineum, and gently guide the knee toward the floor.

Inhaling, straighten that leg out in front, then exhale, bringing the other foot toward the perineum and gently pushing the knee toward the floor.

Keep alternating the movement a few times.

This exercise can also be done in a fluid, continuous flow of movement synchronized with the breath, as described above. If possible, keep the hands placed on the knees to guide them toward the floor, or keep your hands at your side on the floor.

KNEE TO THE SIDE WITH FORWARD BEND

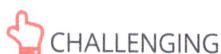

👆 CHALLENGING

Training Focus: Lengthens the muscles of the spine and hamstrings, mobilizes the hip and knee joints.

This more challenging variation of the previous exercise incorporates a forward bend. Do this exercise only if it does not cause you to force or strain.

Sitting with your back straight and your legs stretched out in front of you, use your hand to bring one foot toward your body so that the heel rests at the perineum or at the base of your thigh with the foot pointing down the inner side of the straight leg.

The bent knee rests on or near the floor.

On an exhalation, bend forward from the base of the spine, moving your navel forward and allowing the spine to lengthen.

Without forcing, move forward from the base of your spine in the direction of the knee of the straight leg, bringing your fingers to your toes or your hands to the foot, or shin, or just the knee, depending on what feels right to you at the time. Continue to inhale and exhale calmly and easily.

Go only as far as you can with your back straight. Gradually you will be able to bring your forehead closer to the knee and fingers to the toes.

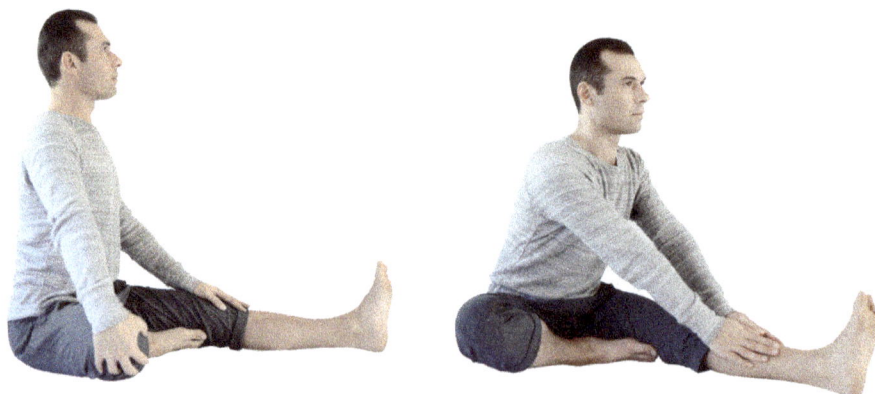

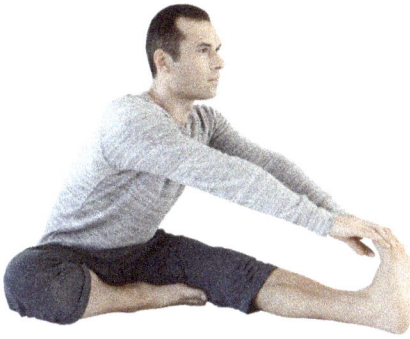

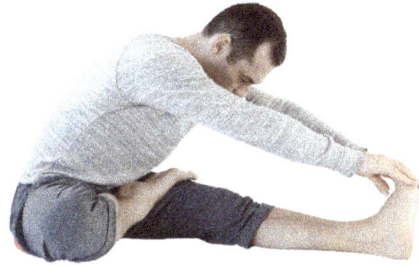

Switch sides and repeat, continuing to alternate the entire sequence on each side a few times.

You can also alternate doing this exercise in a continuous movement and doing it with a static phase while relaxing into the forward bending position.

Once you are sufficiently flexible, you can deepen the stretch by placing your foot on the top of the thigh, at the groin.

ALTERNATE LEG STRETCH

 MODERATE

Training Focus: Lengthens the muscles of the spine and legs.

Sitting with your legs stretched out in front of you, take hold of your toes if possible, or at least your ankles. Keeping the base of the spine stable, point one of your feet forward while exhaling. Then inhale, lengthening your spine, and point the other foot forward as you exhale. Alternate a few times, synchronizing your breathing with the movement.

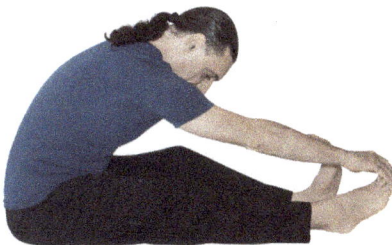

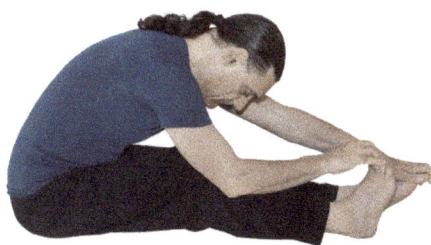

If possible, keep the knee of the leg not being stretched pressing toward the ground. If this is too challenging, let the knee rise a little until you are comfortable, but keep the lower back engaged.

Rather than alternating on each inhalation, you can also stretch one leg at a time, leaning forward on the thigh of the slightly risen inactive leg and leaving the stretched leg firmly on the ground.

CLASSIC FORWARD BEND

👎 CHALLENGING

Training Focus: Stretches the spine and hamstrings. Improves hip flexibility.

Sit with your back straight and your legs stretched out in front of you.

Inhale, raising your arms straight over your head and keeping your spine straight. Exhale, bending forward from the base of the spine, moving your navel forward and allowing your spine to lengthen. Without forcing, try to bring your forehead toward the knees and your fingers to your toes, or to or toward your ankles. Go only as far as you can while making sure to keep your back straight.

Gradually bring your forehead closer to your knees and your fingers closer to your toes.

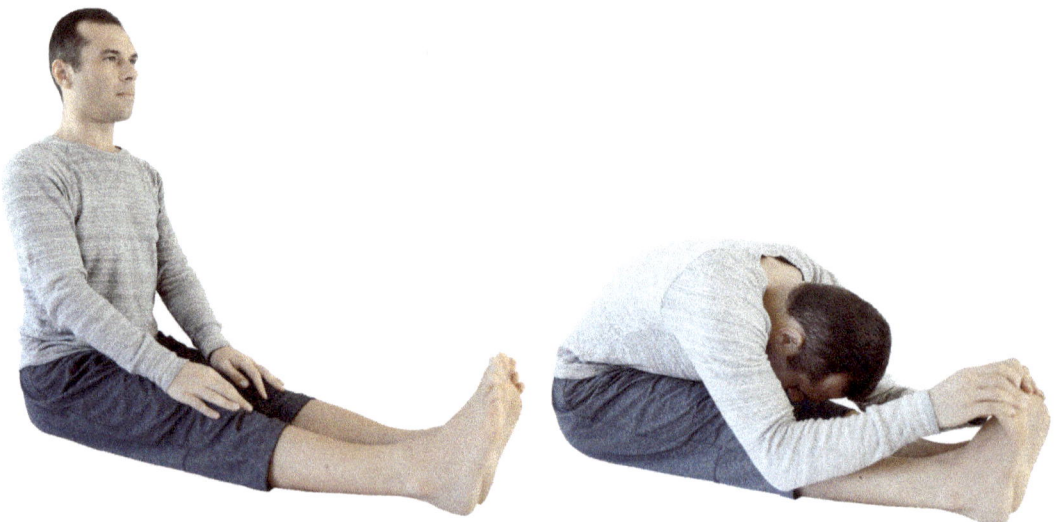

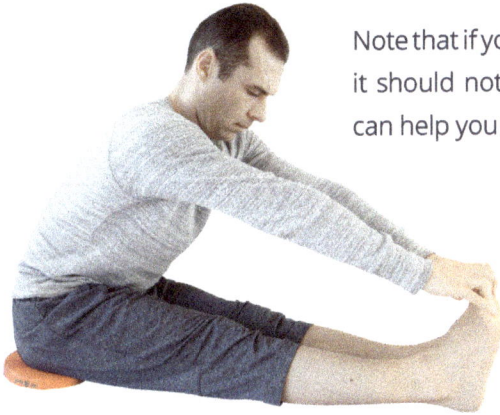

Note that if you use a prop for this kind of exercise, it should not be too thick; often a thinner prop can help you have a better alignment.

BUTTERFLY

👍 MODERATE

Training Focus: Opens the hips and stretches the inner thighs.

Sit with your back straight, your knees open, and the soles of your feet together with your heels close to the perineum. You can sit on a thin prop to ensure better alignment.

Keep your arms stretched along your sides, with your hands or fists on the ground, your shoulders open, and your back straight.

Gently bounce your knees up and down toward the floor, opening your hips as much as possible without straining. Breathe calmly.

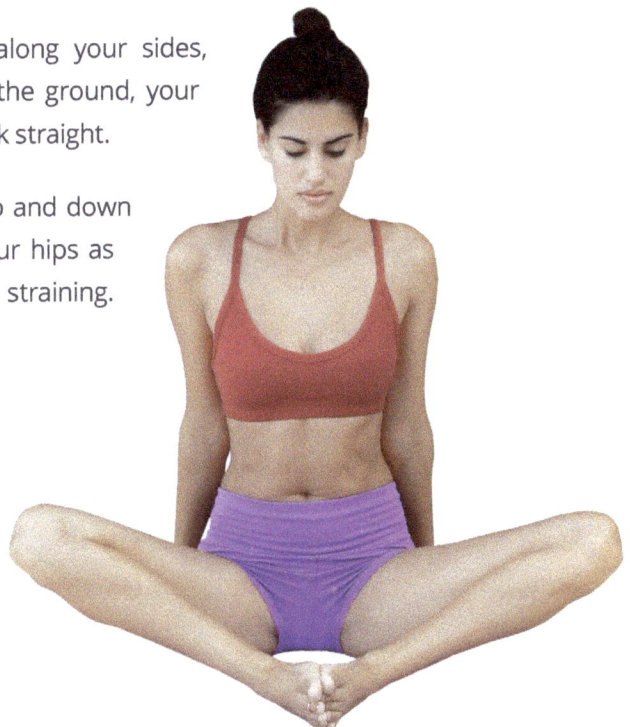

BOTH KNEES TO SIDE FORWARD BEND

Training Focus: Lengthens the spine and mobilizes the hip and knee joints.

This exercise can be done with two different dynamics with respect to the arm movement.

The first one is easier on the lower back. The second is a slightly more challenging version that is even more effective in lengthening the spine, but should definitely not be performed by those with a tender lower back.

Placing a firm prop that is not too thick under your sit bones will make all of these exercises easier.

VERSION I

MODERATE

Sit with one knee to the side and place the heel of the foot at the perineum. Then place the side of the other foot in front, with a distance of two hand spans between the two heels.

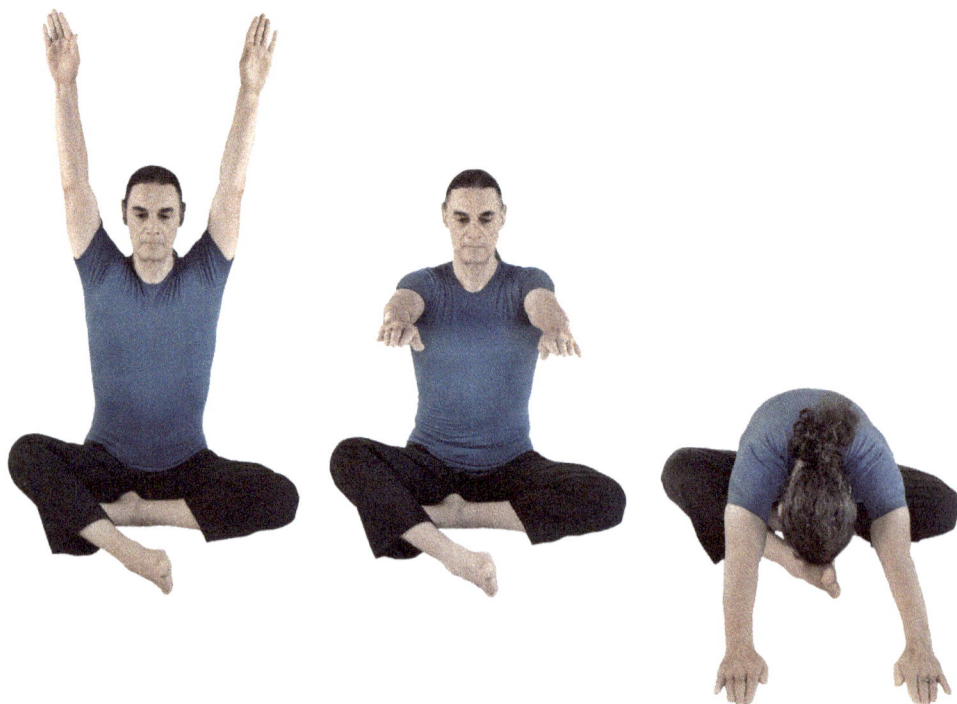

Keeping the back straight, inhale, extending your arms up parallel above the shoulders. Exhaling, bring your arms to shoulder level first, then continue to lower them to or toward the floor as you bend forward, moving your forehead to or toward the arch of the foot.

Now inhale, again extending your arms straight above your shoulders, then exhale, bending forward as before. After a few repetitions you can remain bent forward for a while, breathing calmly and smoothly while holding the position. You can relax your hands out in front or on either side of the front foot.

Remember to stretch from the base of your spine, lengthening and keeping your back straight, but not tense.

Now repeat the entire sequence, reversing the position of your legs, first in motion and then pausing and relaxing in the bent position.

Because in this exercise we first lower the arms to shoulder level, it is quite gentle on the lower back. It is also very effective in relaxing any tension of the spine.

VERSION II

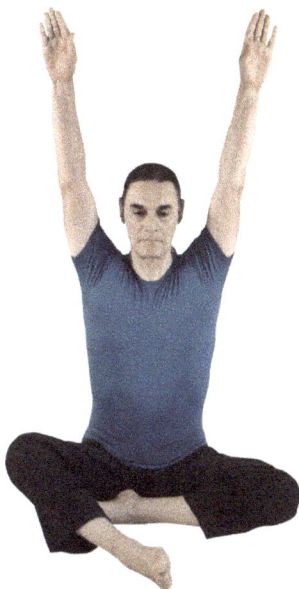 CHALLENGING

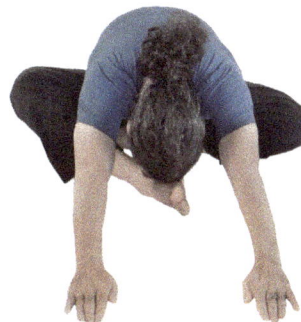

Sit as before, with one foot at the perineum and the other foot in front, with a distance of two hand spans between the two heels, letting the weight of the legs draw the knees toward the floor.

Inhale, extending your arms straight above your shoulders. Then exhale as you bend forward, keeping your arms stretched out in front and bringing the hands toward the floor as you lower your forehead to or toward the arch of the front foot.

Keep the back straight but not tense as you move forward, initiating the movement from the navel, not from the shoulders.

The movement, done in this way, will naturally contribute to thoroughly lengthening your spine.

Now inhale and raise your arms back above your head, first sliding your hands toward the knees and then raising them above your head. Then exhale, bending forward again.

After a few repetitions you can stay bent forward for a while, calmly and smoothly breathing in the position.

Repeat the sequence a few times, then reverse the position of your legs and repeat the entire sequence again.

VERSION III

MODERATE

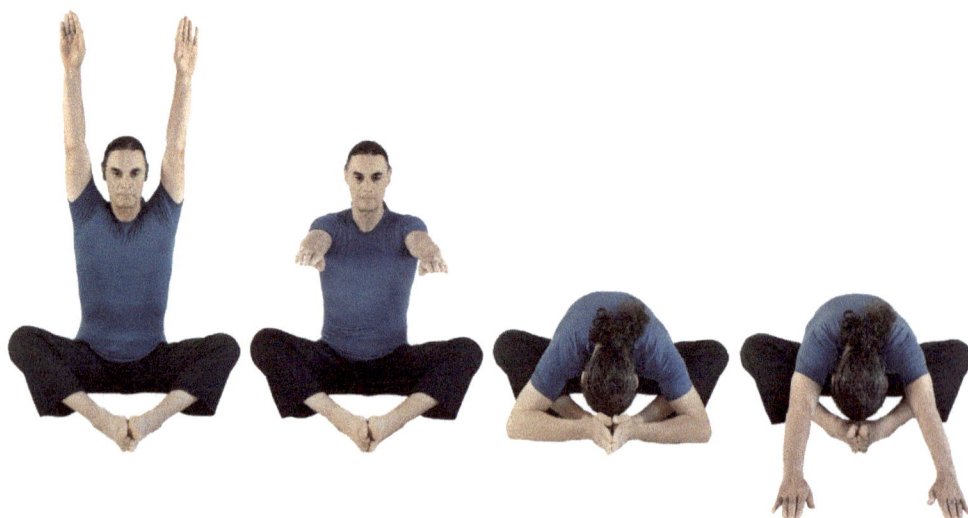

Joining the soles of your feet two hand spans in front of your perineum, repeat the entire sequence as before, first in motion and then pausing and relaxing. Again, you can first lower your arms to shoulder level and bend forward gradually, and then – if your back permits – stretch directly forward with the arms straight and parallel along the sides of the head. Move your forehead to or toward the arches of your feet. You can stretch your arms out in front or hold onto your feet with your hands.

Repeat the sequence a few times without forcing or overdoing it. Exhale bending forward and inhale coming back up.

VERSION IV

 EASY

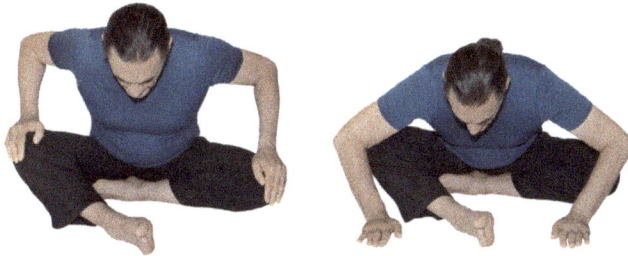

It is also possible to perform the same exercises – with or without the soles of the feet joined – without raising your arms above the head, but simply keeping them on your knees, or in front on the floor, to give you support for the movement.

Inhale as you bend forward and exhale as you rise back up.

TURN AND STRETCH

VERSION I

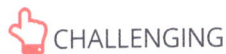CHALLENGING

Training Focus: This exercise is a particularly effective and comprehensive warm-up, and it helps you develop a correct sitting position. It is also highly useful for opening the hips for the lotus and the half-lotus pose.

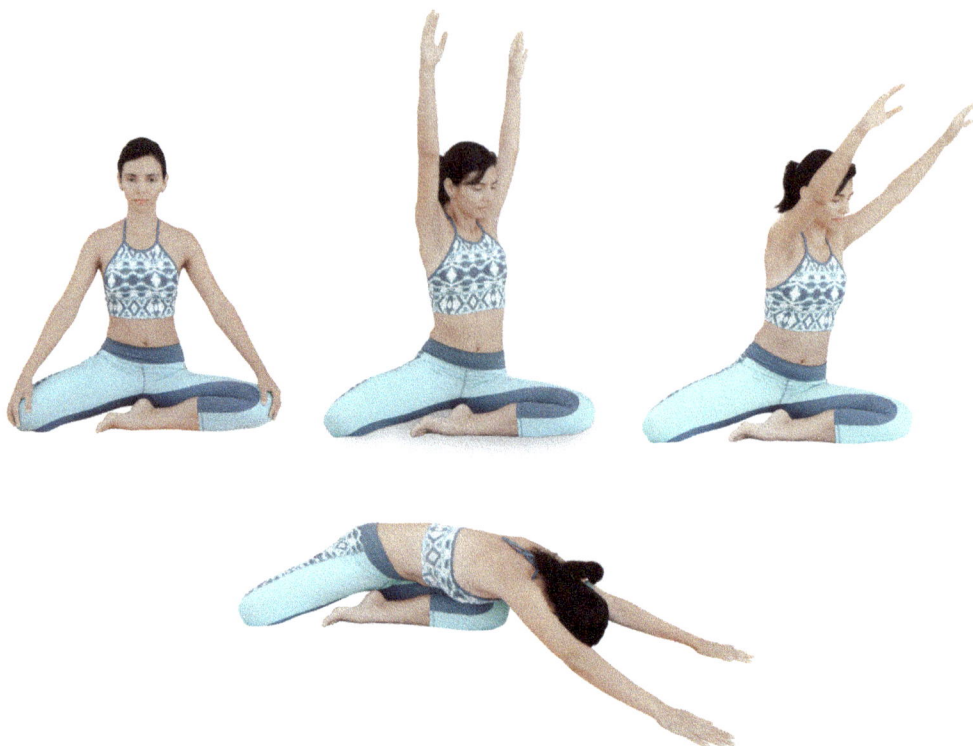

Sit on the floor with one leg bent in front and the heel at your perineum. Bend the other leg behind you, keeping the foot close to your buttocks without sitting on it.

Inhaling, stretch your arms straight up. Then, just before your inhalation is complete, stretch up a bit more and turn from the root of the spine – not from the shoulders – to face the front knee. Be sure not to block your breathing. Keep it open and smooth.

Exhaling, stretch forward and bring your forehead and outstretched hands to or toward the floor in front of that knee.

Inhaling, rise up, straightening the spine, and bring your arms up parallel, extended above the head. Turn to the other side and, to the extent possible, bring your forehead in front of the other knee, extending your arms forward. The forward bend will probably be more difficult on one side. It is important not to force. Instead, gently try to reach forward as far as is comfortable.

Repeat one or two more times.

Reverse the position of your legs and repeat the sequence on the other side.

VERSION II

👍 MODERATE

A slight variation in the dynamics of the movement and the breathing will make the exercise a bit easier, especially for less flexible people or who might have some tenderness in the lower back.

Sit on the floor with one leg bent in front, heel at your perineum, and the other leg behind you, placing the foot as close to your buttocks as possible without sitting on it.

Inhaling, stretch your arms straight up from the shoulders. As you do this the hands face outward.

Be sure not to block your breathing. Keep it open and smooth.

Exhaling, lower your arms to shoulder level, then turn to gradually face the front knee as you bring your outstretched hands to or toward the floor.

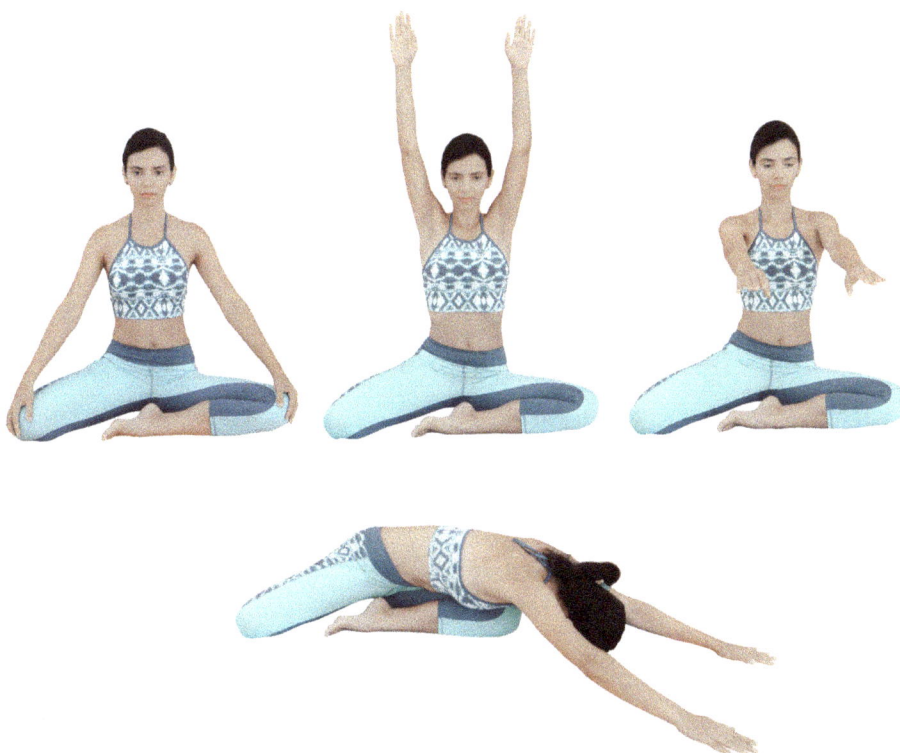

VERSION III

👍 MODERATE

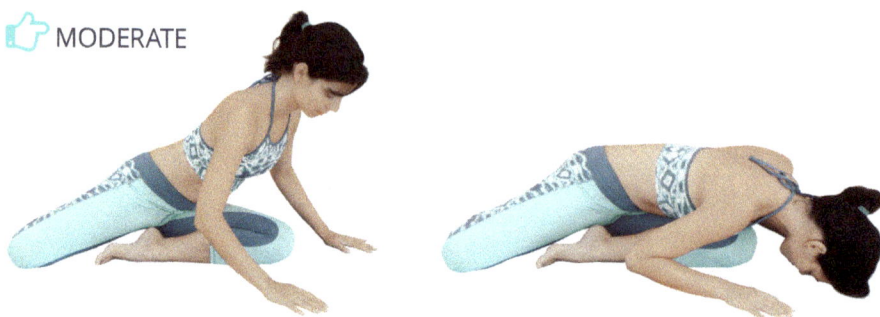

In this third variation, lower your arms to the sides of the front knee first and then lower your head to or toward the floor.

In this way you can support the motion of bending forward and make it more controlled and easier.

KNEE BEND

👍 CHALLENGING

Training Focus: Mobilizes the knee and hip joints.

It is better not to attempt this exercise at the start of a warm-up session. Do it only after the knees have been properly warmed up.

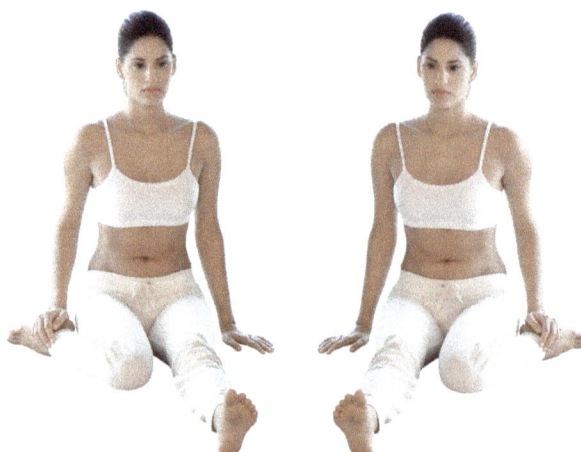

Sit with your legs stretched out in front and your back straight, your hands on the floor at your sides. Inhale smoothly and calmly, and then exhale, leaning slightly to one side and using your hand as a support. At the same time, bend your knee on the other side back and bring the foot to the side, your toes pointing backward close to your body.

As you start to slowly rock your weight to center again, be sure there is no pain in the knee of the bent leg. Otherwise, stop short of bringing the weight all the way to center so that there is less pressure on the bent knee.

Inhale, leaning slightly to the same side as before to help straighten your bent leg forward again. Exhale, repeating the movement on the opposite side. Alternate from side to side in a continuous movement, rocking gently from one sit bone to the other, for three to five sets.

CROSS-KNEE HAMSTRING STRETCH

👆 CHALLENGING

Training Focus: Lengthens the spine and hamstrings, mobilizes the hip and knee joints.

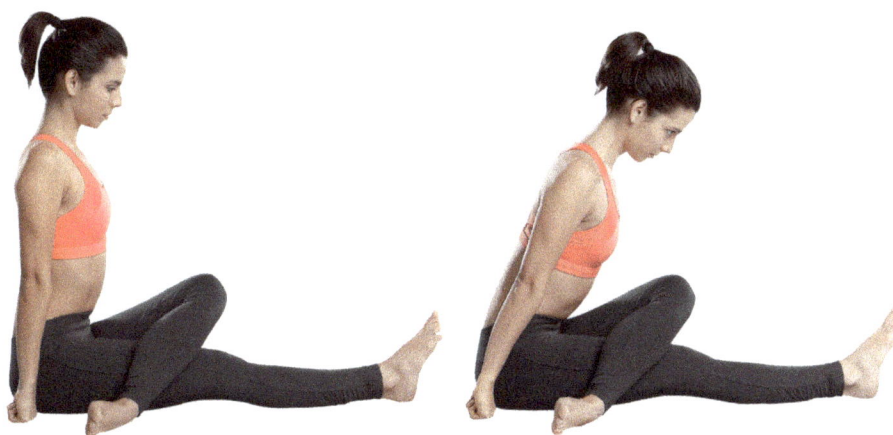

Sitting with one leg extended, cross your other leg over the knee, placing the foot next to your hip. Now, with one knee over the other, place your hand on the upper knee and gently put some weight on it, which helps to straighten the leg under it. Then place your palms or your fists on the floor behind you.

You can make the exercise easier by putting a thin blanket or yoga prop under your sit bones.

Inhale and exhale, alternately pointing and flexing the foot of the outstretched leg a few times.

Now, inhaling in a fluid, calm way, straighten your spine and then exhale, leaning forward over your thigh. Move forward from your navel, not your shoulders, and keep the back straight, without hunching.

Inhale as you move back to the upright position.

It is important to synchronize the movement and breathing.

If you can use the breathing to help the movement, you will need less effort without sacrificing energy or strength.

After repeating this movement a few times, you can add a rest at the end of the forward bending movement. Hold the position, but without holding your breath. Breathe calmly and smoothly.

Very gradually, extend a bit more every time you come forward, always relaxing the breathing into the movement.

Repeat a few times on each side.

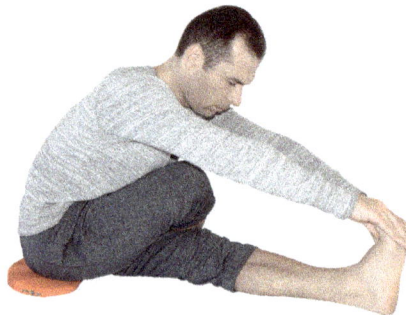

Finally, try to put both hands on the foot of your extended leg.

To increase the effectiveness of the movement, where possible, do all of the above sequences keeping the foot of the extended leg flexed firmly backward.

Pause for a moment, then switch sides and repeat a few times on the other side.

SIDE STRETCH

👍 MODERATE

Training Focus: Stretches the lateral muscles of the spine and legs.

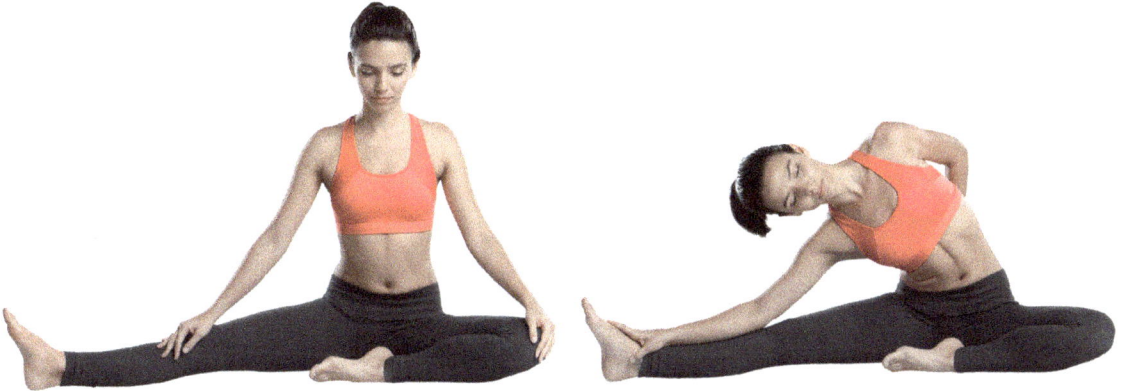

Sit with your back straight and the soles of the feet joined in front, as close to the perineum as possible.

Then stretch one leg wide to the side, placing your hands on your knees. Breathing calmly and smoothly, lean to the side of the outstretched leg and try to bring the corresponding hand to that ankle. If you like you can bring the other hand to your lower back. Hold for a little while, breathing calmly.

Move back to the previous position with the soles of the feet together, then stretch the other leg wide to the side and repeat the same sequence.

Once you are familiar with the dynamics of the exercise you can coordinate the movement with the breathing: Inhale in the starting position, then exhale as you open one leg wide to the side. Leaning to the side without turning your torso, but keeping it as much as possible in the same plane as the open leg, bring your hand to or toward the ankle. Inhale, coming back to the starting position, then exhale as you open the leg to the other side and lean toward it.

Repeat the sequence of movement a few times, always breathing calmly and fully, coordinating the breathing with the movement. Never hold the breath.

RECLINING WARM-UPS

FULL-BODY SHAKE

👍 EASY

Training Focus: Loosens the arm and leg joints.

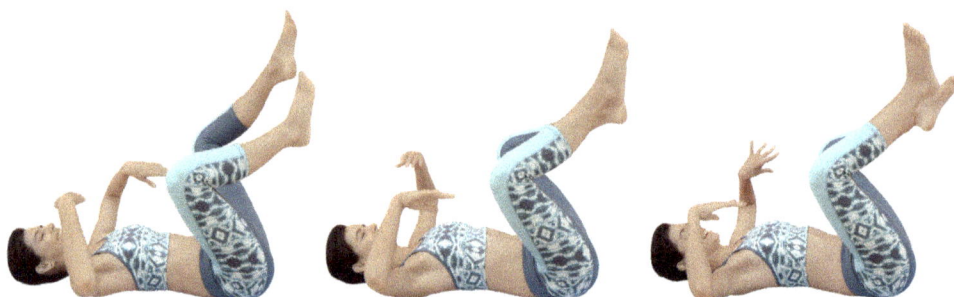

Lying on your back, shake all limbs freely and vigorously. Breathe spontaneously and enjoy the sensation of release.

KNEE TO CHEST

Training Focus: Mobilizes and relaxes the muscles of the hips and back. Helps keep the lower back healthy.

VERSION I

👍 EASY

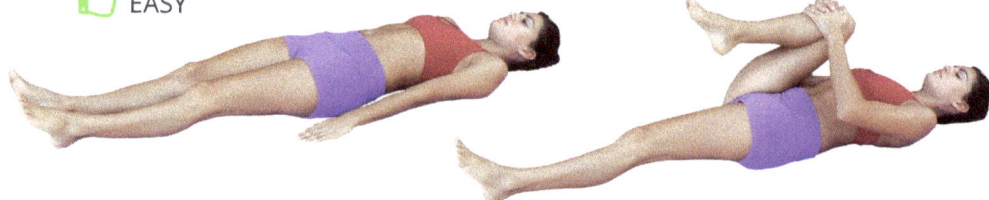

Lying on your back, exhale as you bring one knee toward your chest, clasping it with both hands. Then inhale, stretching your leg along the floor again, keeping it fully extended and straight.

Exhale as you bring your other knee toward your chest, and then inhale as you extend your leg back along the floor. Switch sides and repeat, alternating the sequence three to five times.

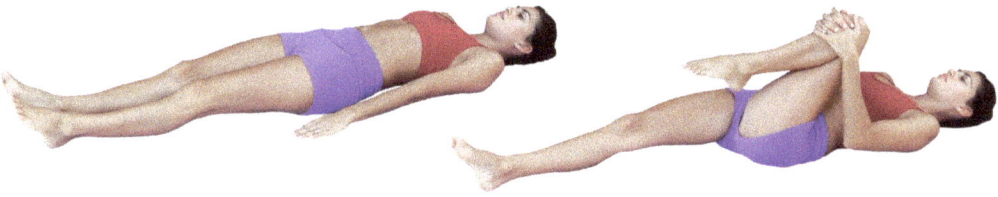

VERSION II

👉 MODERATE

For a slightly more challenging alternative, you can do the same exercise keeping your extended leg just off the floor, vigorously controlled with the foot pointed, while you hug the other knee to the chest. Inhaling, bring the other knee toward the chest until joins the first knee, then exhale and extend the other leg.

Alternate the sequence a few times.

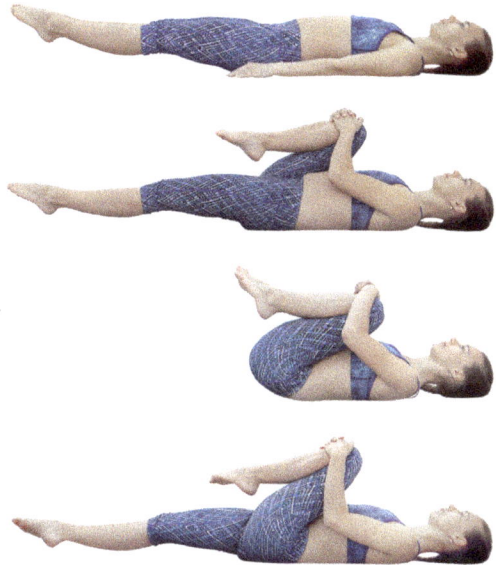

VERSION III

👉 CHALLENGING

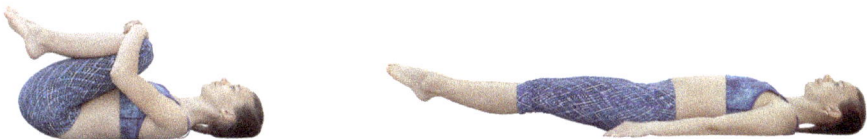

Finally, if you feel comfortable, you can stretch both legs forward, keeping them controlled with your feet about a hand width off the floor.

Hold the position for about ten counts. Then, on an exhalation, bring the knees back to the chest. Repeat five to fifteen times.

With each exhalation, pull your knees a bit closer to your chest.

PERPENDICULAR LEG STRETCH

👍 EASY

Training Focus: Mobilizes the knee and hip joints while releasing tension in the lower abdomen.

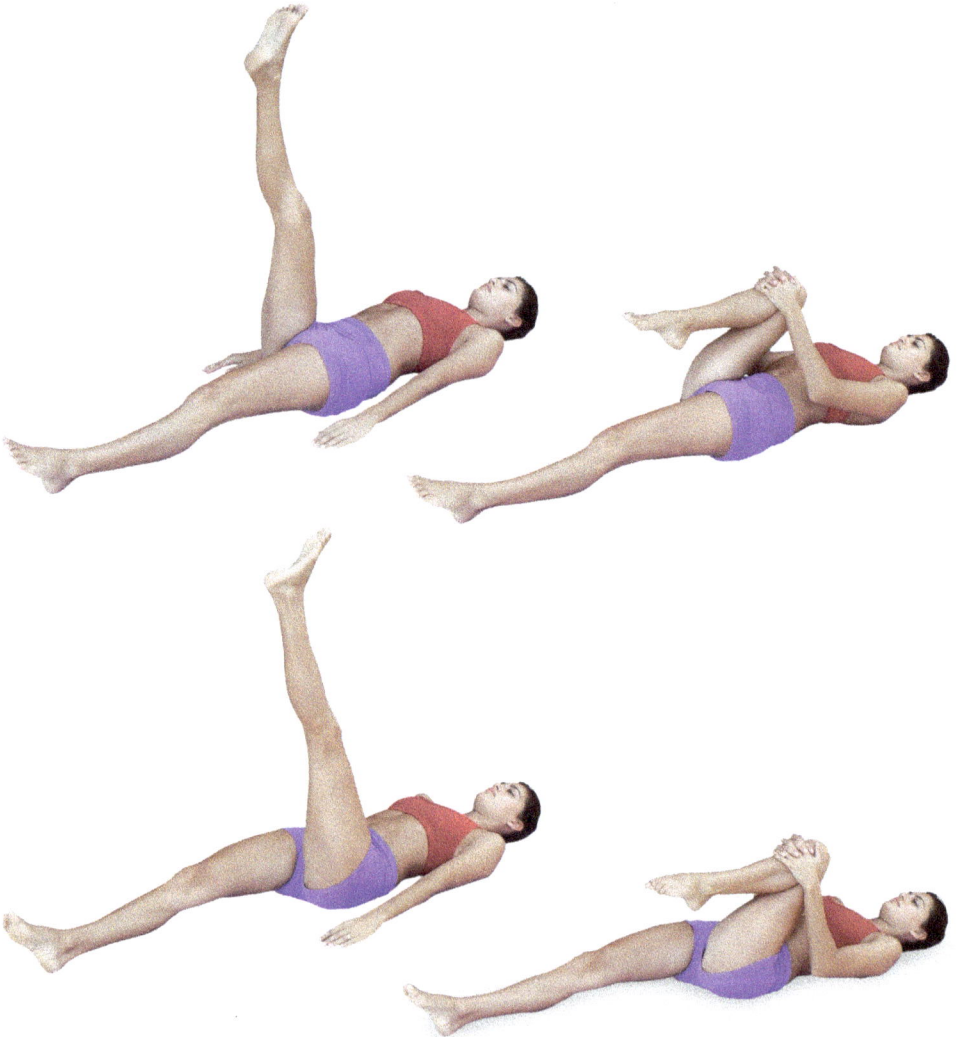

Lying on your back, inhale and extend one leg straight up. Exhale as you bend the leg and bring the knee to your chest, clasping it with both hands. Inhale, extending your leg straight up again, and then exhale as you lower the leg to the floor.

Switch sides and repeat, continuing to alternate the entire sequence a few times.

SUPINE TWIST

👍 MODERATE

Training Focus: Improves flexibility of the spine while increasing awareness of abdominal, intercostal, and dorsal breathing.

This exercise uses a simple and safe twist that is especially effective for maintaining a healthy back.

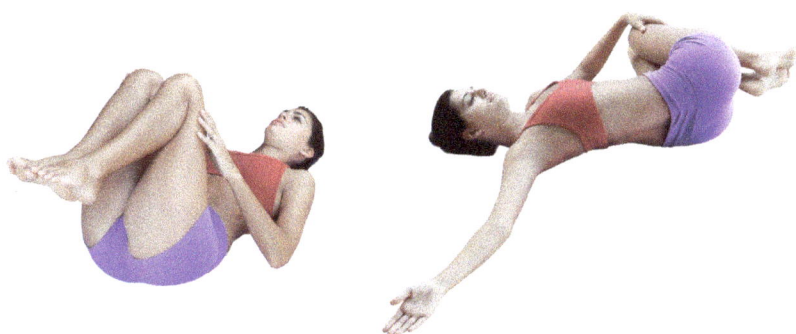

Lying on your back, bring your knees to the chest and then roll onto one side with your knees and feet as close together as possible, one on top of the other.

Inhaling, open and stretch your top arm wide to the side, keeping your shoulders and knees on the floor.

If you find opening your arm to the side difficult you can bring your hand to the shoulder or place it on the chest instead. You can also place your outstretched hand on a pillow or any props to support it. If the twist feels too challenging, you can put a small pillow under the lower knee.

Keep the head centered, breathing calmly and smoothly as you relax in the pose.

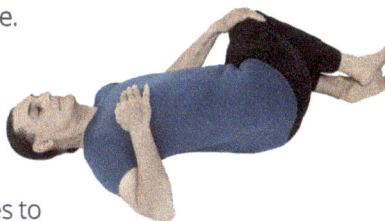

Now roll back to the center with both knees to the chest, then onto the other side to repeat the exercise. Continue to alternate a few times.

OUTER THIGH STRETCH

👍 MODERATE

Training Focus: Stretches the rotator muscles of the hips. Also effective for opening your hips for the lotus pose. Good for the lower back.

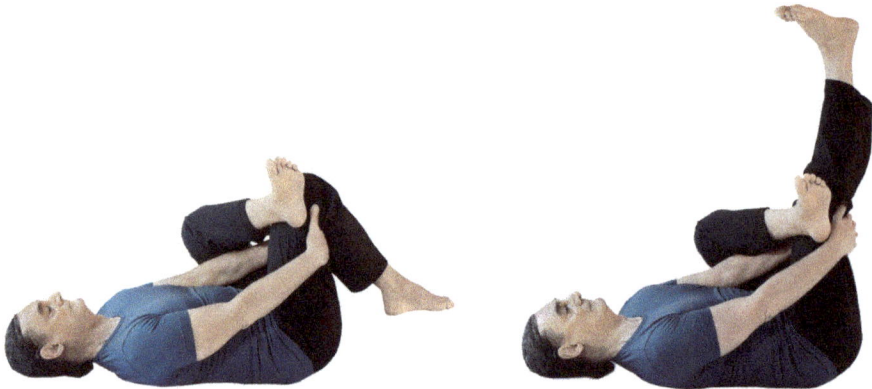

Lying on your back with your knees toward the chest, place one foot on the other thigh, just above the knee. Then reach inside the space between your legs with one hand and around the back thigh with the other to interlace your fingers behind the thigh, near the knee.

On an exhalation gently pull the leg toward the chest, then, while inhaling, ease the tension of the pull, and exhaling pull it toward the chest again. Or, if you prefer, you can keep the leg pulled toward the chest.

After some time in this position, raise the back leg straight up while inhaling and flexing your foot. As you exhale, bend the knee again to bring the leg back down.

Repeat this a few times then switch to the other side and repeat the sequence.

GENTLE CRUNCH

Training Focus: Strengthens the abdominal muscles.

VERSION I

👍 MODERATE

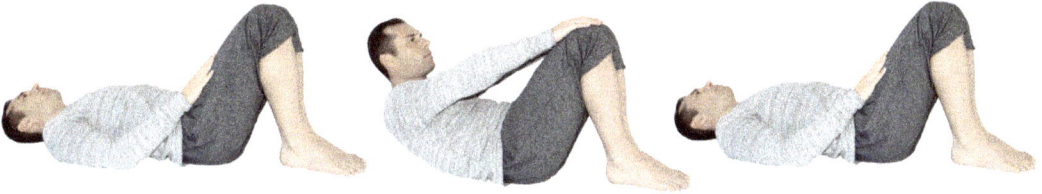

This is a gentle, safe, and effective exercise for training the abdominal muscles. It is simple and quite commonly used in many different disciplines. Training and toning the abdominal muscles is important not only for physical strength but also for cultivating a healthier breathing pattern.

Lie on your back and bend your knees to bring the heels close to the sit bones.

Put your hands on your thighs and – keeping your feet on the floor – slide your hands up the thighs to bring them to or toward the knees or the sides of the knees as you lift the shoulders and upper back off the floor. Hold briefly, then relax back down.

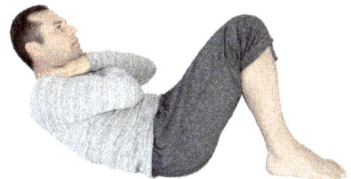

Repeat this action three, five, or more times.

VERSION II

👍 MODERATE

For a variation, cross your arms at the chest and hold onto your shoulders. Keeping your feet on the floor close to the sit bones, lift your shoulders and upper back off the floor, hold briefly, then relax back down.

VERSION III

👆 CHALLENGING

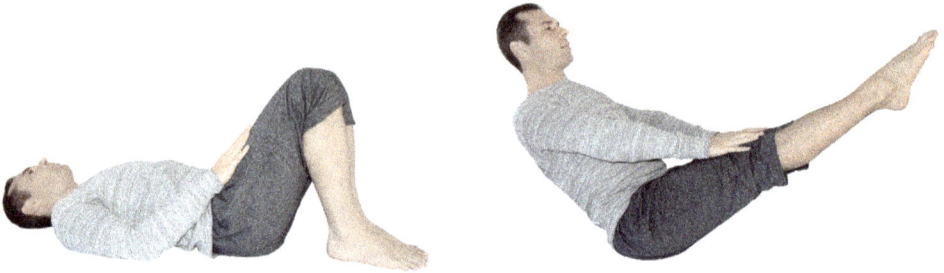

In yet another variation, you rise off the floor with both your torso end legs firmly engaged: To begin, lying on the floor with your heels close to your sit bones, place your hands on your thighs and as you inhale slide them up to reach the knees. Straighten the legs and back into the shape of a triangle for a moment before exhaling and relaxing on the floor.

Repeat a few times.

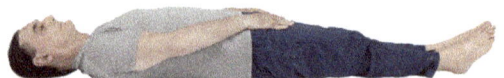

LEG RAISES

👆 CHALLENGING

Training Focus: Strengthens the abdominal muscles, leg muscles, and lower back.

Lie on the floor and rest your hands on your thighs.

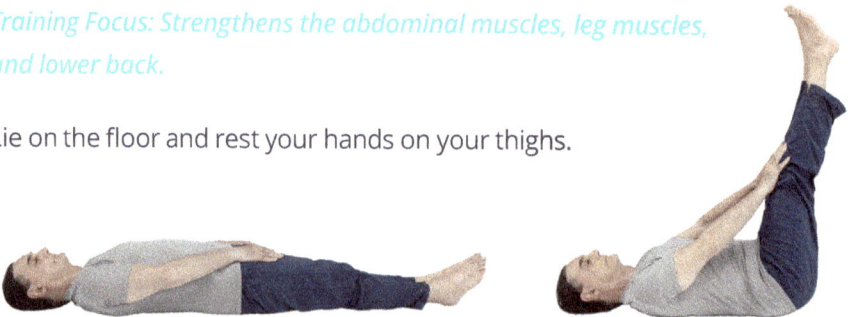

Inhaling, slide the hands along the thighs while raising your legs straight up. Then exhale as you gently lower your legs back to the floor.

Repeat a few times.

THE BRIDGE

Training Focus: Releases tension in the spine and makes it more flexible.

VERSION I: BASIC BRIDGE

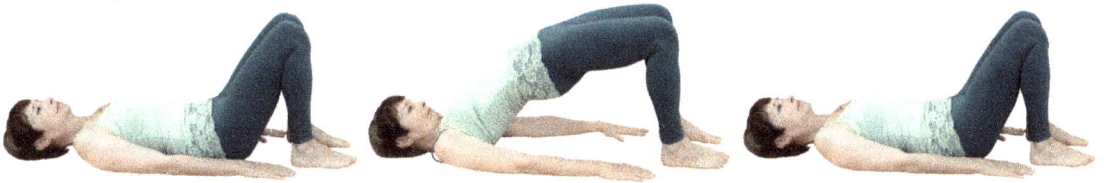

👍 EASY

Lie on your back with your heels close to your sit bones and your arms along your sides. Inhaling, raise your hips into the air as you gently lift your lower back up and off the floor. Then exhale, rolling your spine back down to the floor. Repeat the sequence three to five times, arching upward a little more with each new inhalation, but without forcing, consciously coordinating the continuous flow of the movement of your body with the flow of your breath. Exhale gently and rest for a few moments on the floor. Repeat the sequence as a continuous movement coordinated with the breathing.

You can also try incorporating a conscious **pelvic tilt** when you do the Basic Bridge. Aside from bringing more strength and awareness to your pelvic floor area in general, it improves bladder control and function and reduces the risk of prolapse of internal organs.

Start by lying on your back with your heels close to your sit bones and your arms along the sides. Press your lower back into the floor and, on an inhalation, tilt your pelvis toward your navel as you gently lift the lower back up and off the floor. Firm the buttocks (without hardening) as you lift the hips up. Then exhale, roll your spine back down to the floor, and release the pelvis away from your navel.

When you lift your hips, do not lift them so high that your back arches. Keep your body in a straight line. Gently squeezing your buttock muscles relieves some of the tension from your lower back muscles.

VERSION II: OPEN BRIDGE

👍 EASY

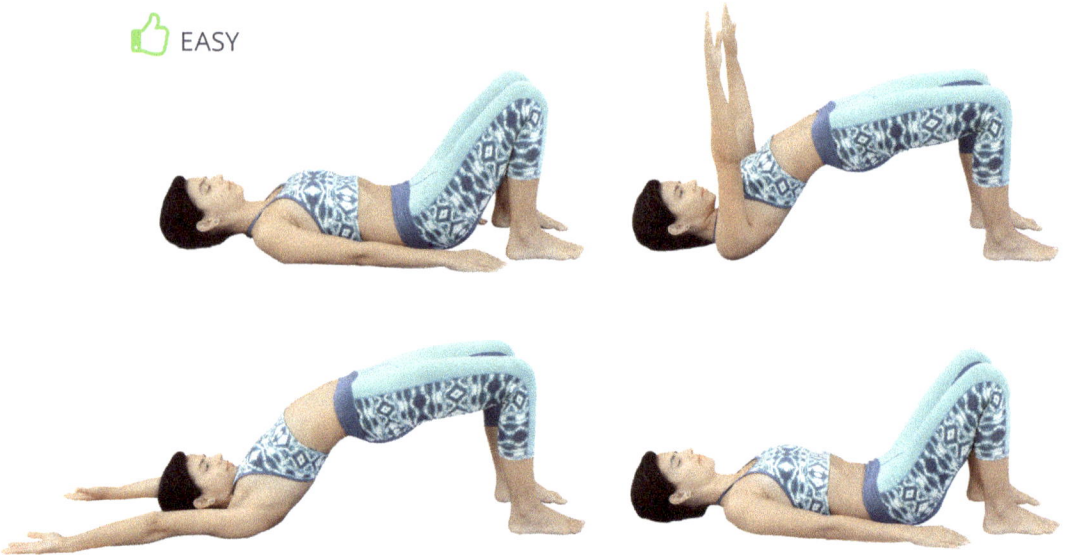

This variation on the Basic Bridge is one of the exercises to develop abdominal breathing.

Unlike in the Basic Bridge, this time, as you inhale and lift your hips up to arch your back, stretch your arms straight up and over your head to the floor.

The arc described by the arms, the arching of the back, and the flow of the breath should all happen simultaneously and be harmoniously synchronized.

Now exhale, raising your extended arms directly above your eyes and then slowly bringing your hands to the ground on either side of the hips as you gradually lower the spine to the ground. To increase the experience of exhaling from the top first, you can join your hands when you start the exhalation. Coordinate the movement with smooth, calm breathing. At this point, if needed, you may want to relax for one or two breathing cycles before repeating the exercise no more than five times.

FACE-DOWN WARM-UPS

LOCUST TRAINING

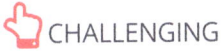

👍 CHALLENGING

Training Focus: Strengthens and tones the muscles of the lower back and buttocks.

Lie on your stomach with your chin on the floor and your arms along your sides. Or, for an easier variation, put your hands under your thighs, palms up.

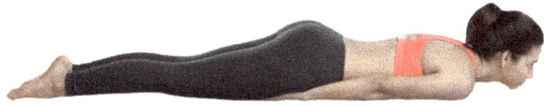

Inhaling, raise one leg up, keeping it taut and straight with the foot pointed. Try to not to bend your knee or open and rotate your hip.

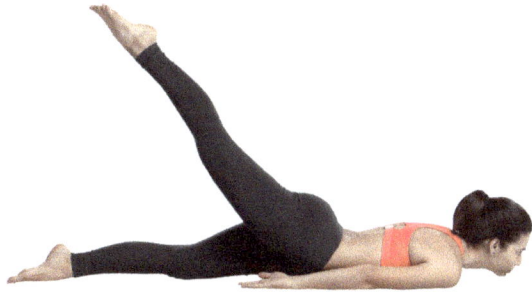

Exhaling, lower your leg back to the floor.

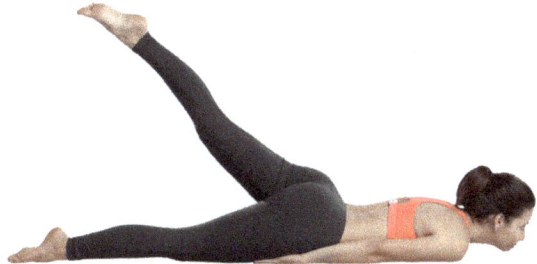

Repeat the action on the other side, continuing to alternate legs a few times.

If you want to go easy on your neck, you may want to perform this pose with your forehead resting on your crossed arms or on your hands in front of you.

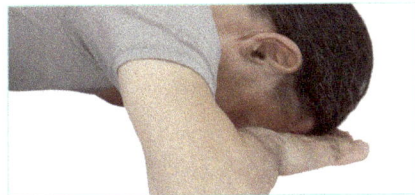

FACE-DOWN HIP OPENER

Training Focus: Particularly effective for opening the hips for the lotus position. Improves hip and knee joint flexibility.

VERSION I: BASIC

👎 CHALLENGING

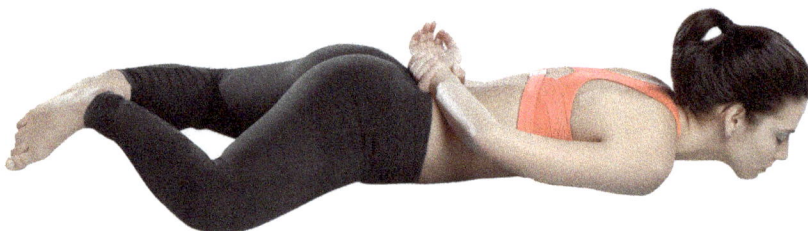

Lie on your stomach with your chin on the floor and arms along the side. Spread your knees open while placing the soles of the feet together and keeping the navel on the floor.

An alternate way to get into the pose is start with the head face down. Position the knees, feet, and hands as described above, and only then lift the head enough to place the chin on the ground.

Clasp your hands behind your back and gradually bring your feet to or toward the floor without separating them. Stay here for a few breaths.

As with the previous exercise, if you want to go easy on your neck, you can also do this exercise with your forehead resting on your crossed arms or on your hands in front of you.

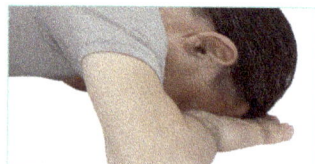

VERSION I: DYNAMIC

👎 CHALLENGING

Enter the position as in Version I. Now inhale, opening your legs wide, then exhale, joining your feet and bringing them back toward the floor. Repeat three to five times.

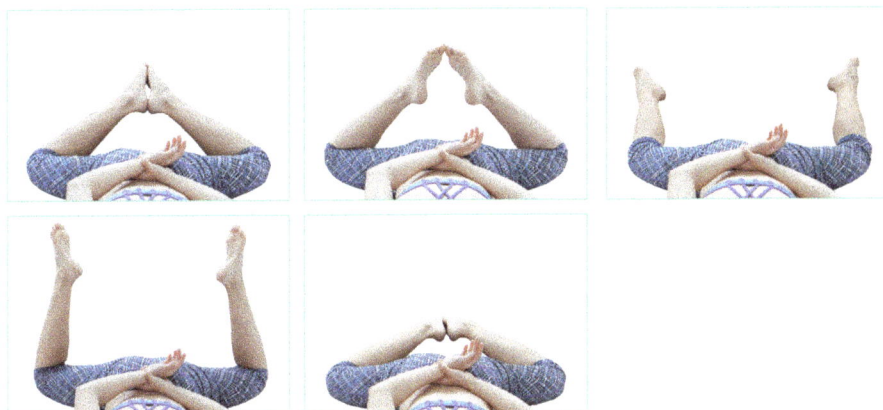

SNAKE TRAINING I

👍 MODERATE

Training Focus: Strengthens back and stomach muscles. Mobilizes the spine.

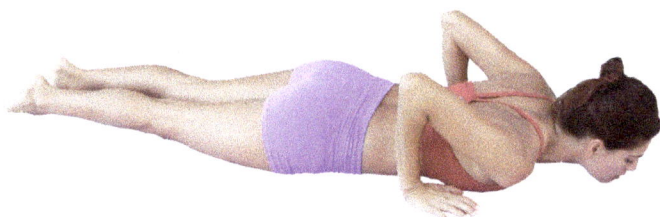

Lie face down with your chin or your forehead on the floor and your hands at chest level or, to make it easier, a bit further toward the head.

Inhaling slowly and gently, raise your torso up and slightly arch your head back, trying, if possible, to keep your spine long and the arms straight.

Exhaling, bring your forehead back to the floor.

Keep your movements slow and coordinated.

Repeat a few times.

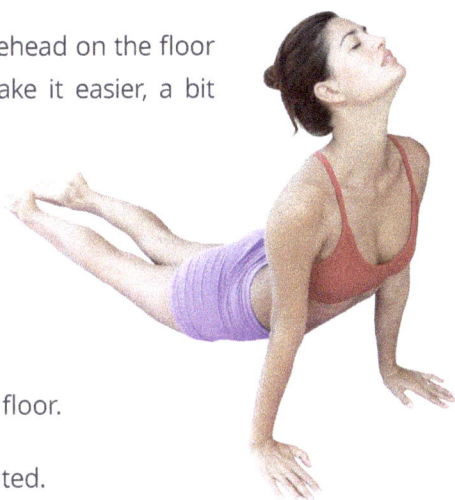

SNAKE TRAINING II

👆 CHALLENGING

Training Focus: Opens the shoulders and increases flexibility of the spine and hips.

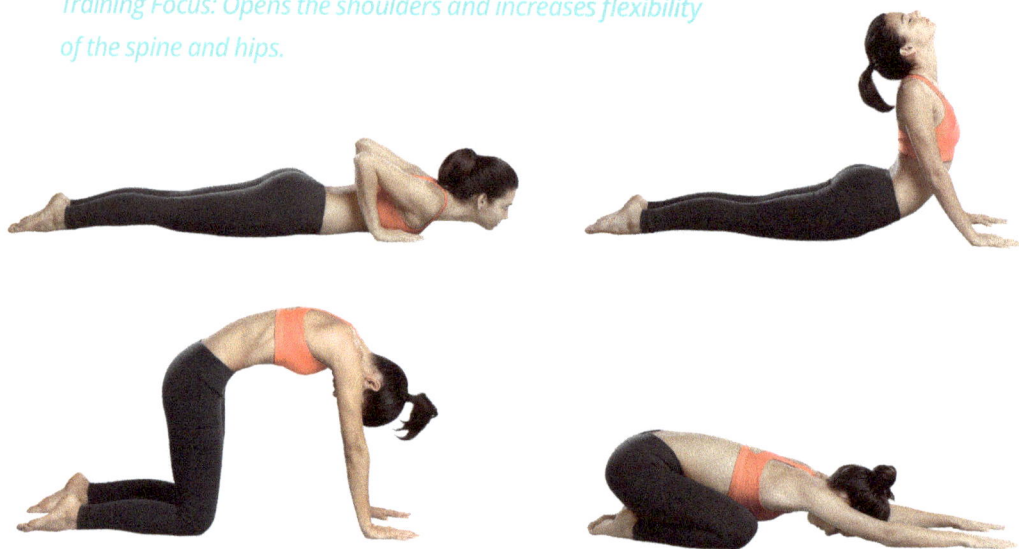

Lie on your stomach with your chin or your forehead on the floor and your hands alongside the mid-level of your chest.

Inhaling, keep your palms on the floor while arching your head back and straightening your arms as much as possible.

Exhaling, counterarch your back and come to sit on your heels, keeping your hands in the same position on the floor.

Now inhale and come to all fours.

Then exhale, lying down with your forehead on the floor again. Repeat the entire sequence three to five times.

SNAKE TRAINING III

👍 CHALLENGING

Training Focus: Mobilizes the spine and hip joints.

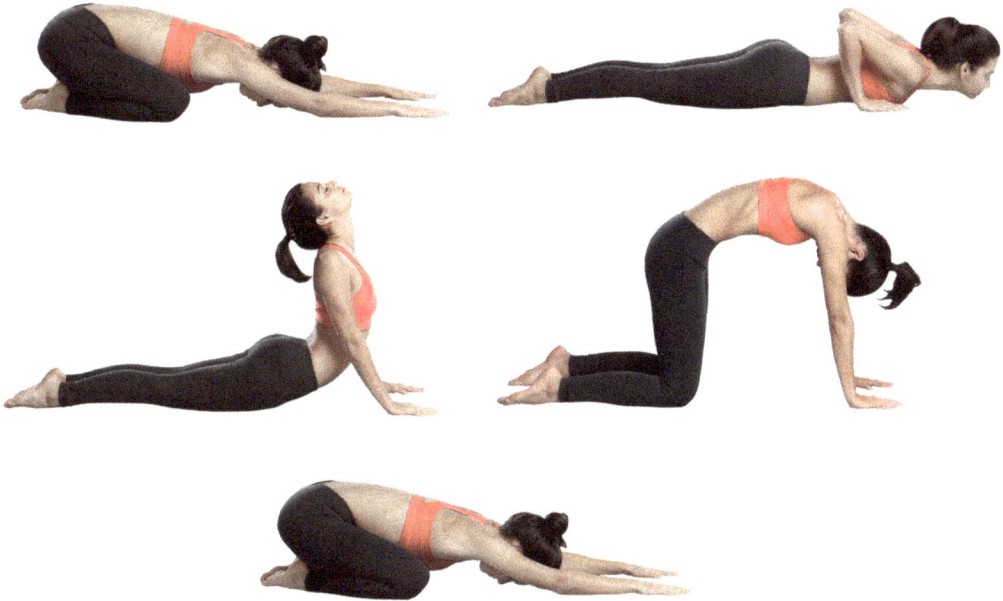

From a kneeling position, stretch your hands to the floor in front of you and place your forehead on the floor as well. Keeping your palms in the same position, inhale as you slide your torso straight forward along the ground, place your chin on the floor, and arch your upper body back while trying to keep your lower pubis or upper thighs on the floor.

Exhaling, counterarch to bring your buttocks back to your heels and your forehead to the floor between your arms.

Repeat the movements a few times, in an easy flow of movement and coordinated breathing.

THE CAT

👍 EASY

Training Focus: Mobilizes the spine, hips, and shoulders.

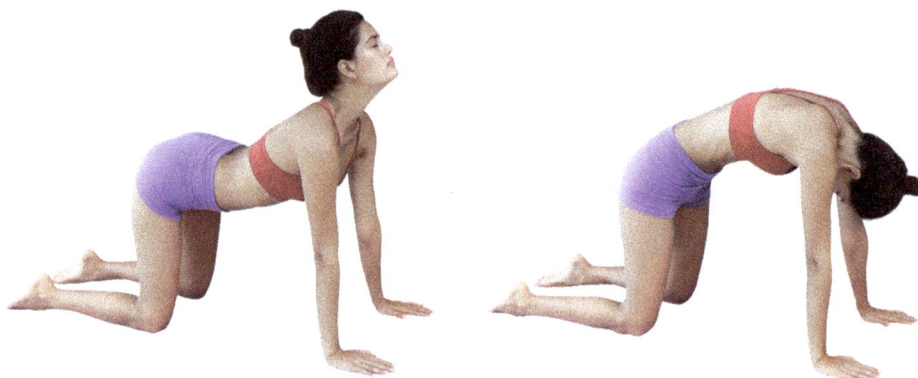

Come onto all fours with your knees a shoulder width apart and your hands directly beneath your shoulders, parallel to your thighs, keeping your arms straight and supporting yourself either on your palms or your fists. Keep the tops of your feet flat on the floor.

Inhaling, lower your navel, bringing your pelvis parallel to the floor while arching your head back and keeping your shoulders as open as possible.

Exhaling, bring your pelvis perpendicular to the floor, curving your mid-back upward, like a cat, and bringing your head between your arms and your chin toward your chest.

Repeat the sequence a few times, maintaining a continuous flow of movement and breathing without ever holding your breath.

It is important not to block the breathing; let it flow freely with the rhythm of the movement.

NECK AND SHOULDER WARM-UPS

Both of these exercises can also be done at the beginning of a warm-up session, either sitting or standing. However, avoid doing them standing if you tend to have low blood pressure.

NECK ROLL

👍 EASY

Training Focus: Improves flexibility of the neck muscles.

All warm-ups should be done calmly and with attention, without forcing the movement or the breathing. This is particularly true here, especially if you have a tender neck.

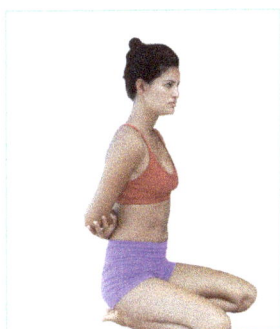

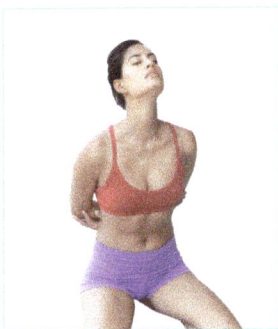

Sitting on your heels, bring your arms behind your back and take hold of your forearms above the elbows. If this is not possible or simply uncomfortable, hold onto one of your wrists.

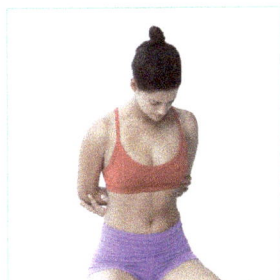

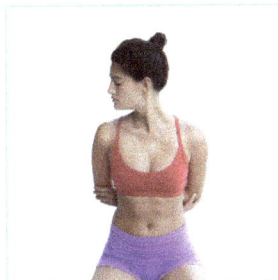

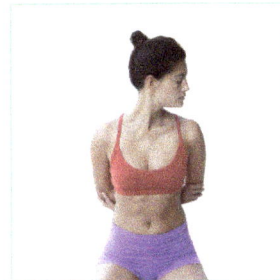

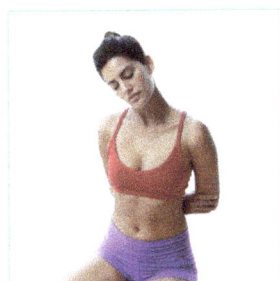

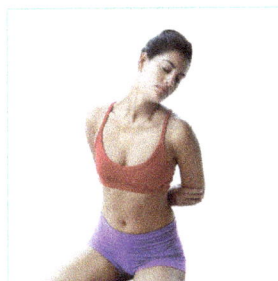

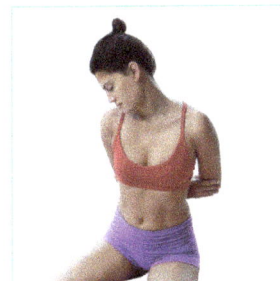

Inhale, arching your head back by stretching your chin up, and then exhale, bringing your chin toward your chest. Move without forcing, slowly and smoothly, keeping your back straight and stable. Repeat one to three times.

Then move to the second phase: With your head centered, inhale and then exhale, turning your head gently but fully to the side. Inhale, moving your head back to the center, then exhale, turning your head to the other side.

To make it softer, you can move your head slightly up when inhaling toward the center and gently down when exhaling and turning to the other side.

Repeat one to three times and then move to the next phase: Exhale, moving one ear toward a shoulder. Inhale, raising your head back to the center, then exhale, bringing your other ear toward your other shoulder. Repeat one to three times.

Then move to the last phase: Inhale, rotating your head to the side and back, then exhale, rotating your head back to the front and bringing your chin to or toward the chest. Repeat, first turning in one direction one to three times, then reversing the rotation and turning the same number of times in the other direction to end the exercise.

MOBILIZING THE SHOULDERS

👍 EASY

Training Focus: Mobilizes the shoulder joints and muscles of the shoulders.

Sitting on your heels with the knees comfortably apart, bring your hands to the top of your shoulders. Inhale, then exhaling, join your elbows in front of your chest. Inhaling, open your elbows up and rotate your shoulders back. Exhaling, bring your elbows down in a circular direction and join them in front again.

Repeat a few times.

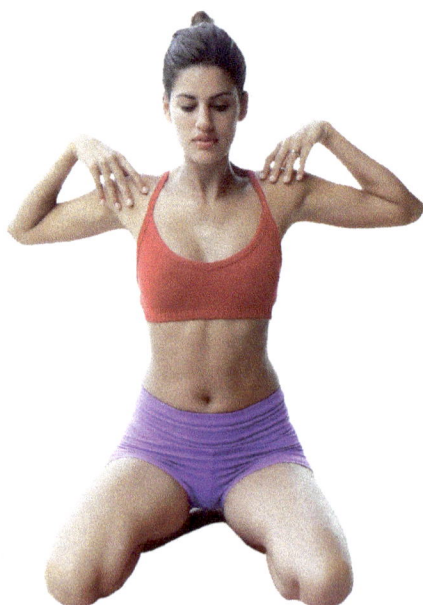

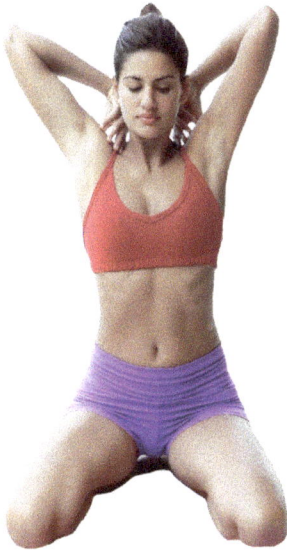

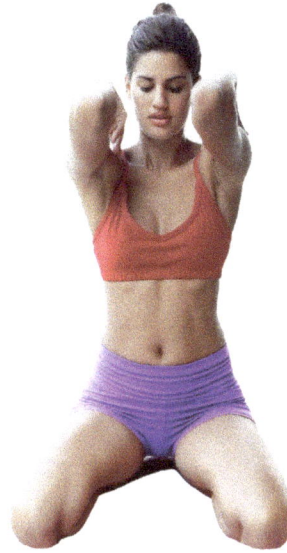

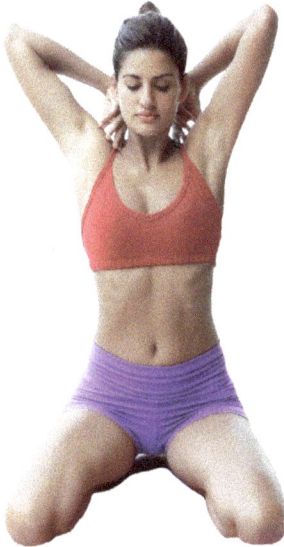

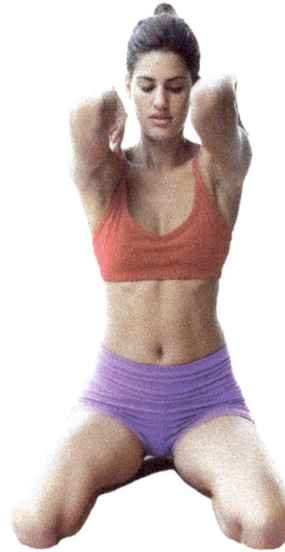

Then inhale as you rotate your elbows in the opposite direction and exhale, joining your elbows at the chest, repeating as in the first direction.

Lastly, alternate the rotation of the movement, doing one rotation in each direction and coordinating each rotation with the corresponding phase of breathing.

Breathe without forcing, but with intent and energy.

It is also possible to do this warm-up without coordinating each phase with the breathing, but simply breathing freely while rotating.

APPENDIX 2 |

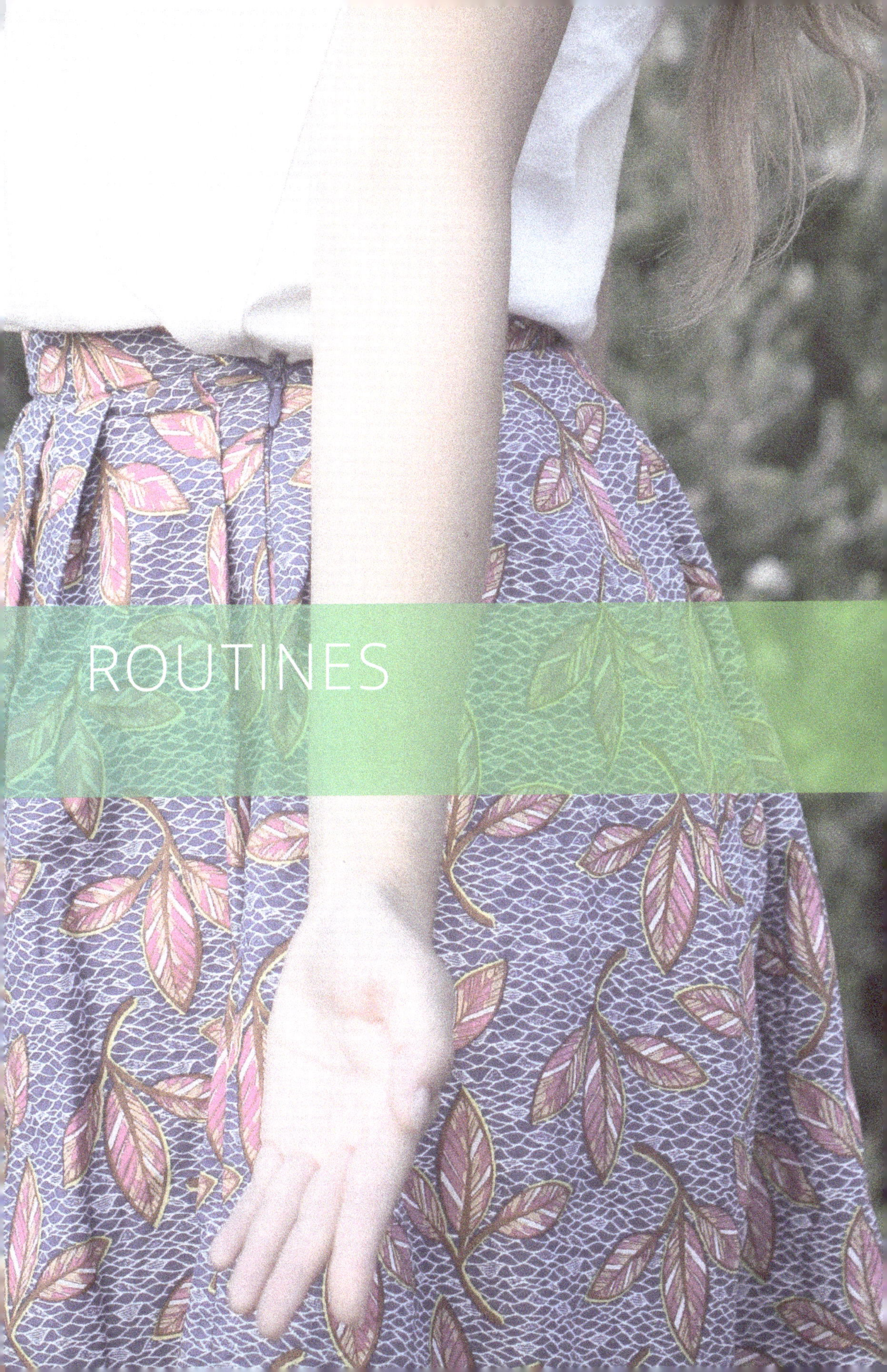

ROUTINES

ROUTINES

Once you are familiar with the basic Harmonious Breathing exercises, you can do a practice session linking a selection of exercises in a sequence. You can create your own routine or follow one of the suggestions given here.

To put together your own routine, the main factors to consider are the amount of time you have available, your level of flexibility, and your personal preferences. For instance, if you have time for a long session, you could do all of the exercises in this book, starting with all or most of the warm-ups and then following the Harmonious Breathing exercises in the sequence given. For a medium session, leave out the ones you find less appealing. Leave out a few more for a short routine. Finally, for a very short practice, choose only three or four of the most crucial exercises.

You could choose only those exercises that can be done with the aid of props, only the "passive" exercises, only dynamic exercises, or a mixture of the two. If you have the opportunity, doing multiple short sessions in the course of a day can be particularly beneficial.

The biggest advantage of creating your own personal routine is that it will include the exercises suited to your condition, the ones you enjoy most, and the ones you find most useful for developing your capacity of complete breathing.

But just to get you started, here are a few examples of different routines.

FULL BREATHING ACTIVATION: 7-MINUTE ROUTINE

Purification Breathing

1 round

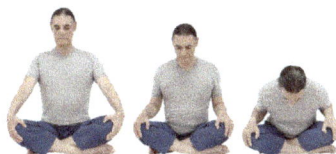

Abdominal Phase

Chin Tuck, sitting or standing: 3 rounds

Four Keys

First Key: Abdominal to Intercostal: 3 rounds
Second Key: Intercostal to Chest: 3 rounds
Third Key: Chest to Upper Chest: 3 rounds
Fourth Key: Collarbone: 3 rounds

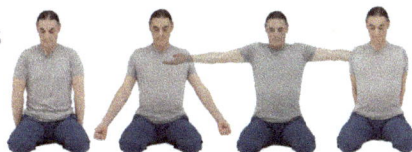

Exhaling from Top to Bottom

Alternative Sequence: 3 rounds

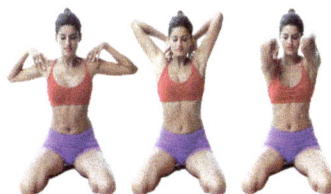

Coordinating the Four Phases

Inhaling Slowly: 3 rounds each

Down, Up, and Arch: 3 rounds each

Coordinating Cat: 3 rounds each

Coordinating Bridge: 3 rounds each

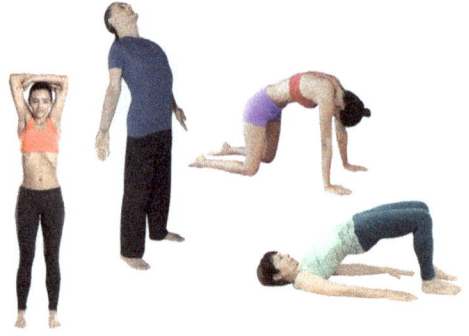

Relaxed, complete respiration

in any seated position: 3 rounds

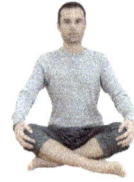

Rhythmic Breathing

(with rhythm 4-6-6): 3 rounds

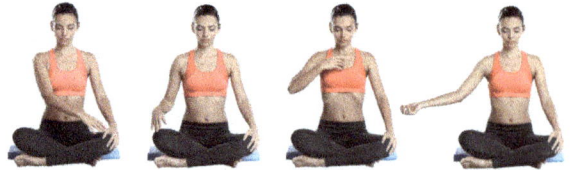

Relaxed, complete respiration

in any seated position, with brief empty
pause after exhalation: 3 rounds

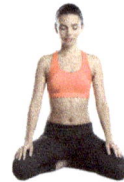

Complete Relaxation

mindful of the flow of the breath: 1 minute

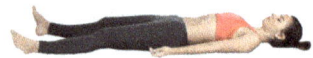

OPEN, COORDINATE, AND RELAX: 10–12-MINUTE PASSIVE ROUTINE

Breathing awareness

any recommended seated position; simply observe and discover the flow of your respiration: 1 minute

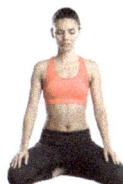

Relax, Open, and Discover

Exercise 1: **Supine Twist**: 2 minutes

Exercise 2: **Resting Dove**: 2 minutes

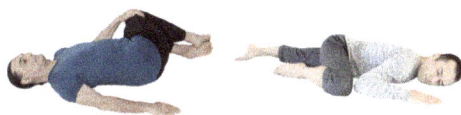

Unifying the Flow

(seated): 1 minute

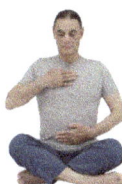

Abdominal Phase

Exercise 3 **(Open Bridge)**: 5 rounds

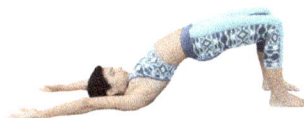

Unifying the Flow

(on floor with open or closed knees): 2 minutes

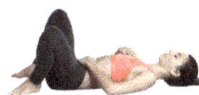

Complete Relaxation

1–3 minutes

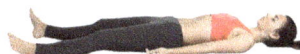

DYNAMIC ENERGIZATION: 12–15-MINUTE ROUTINE

Warm-Ups

Swinging: 3–5 reps

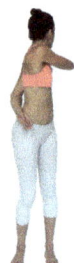

Shaking the Feet:
3–5 reps each side

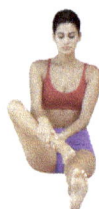

Swinging the Lower Legs:
3–5 reps each side

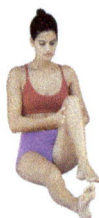

Butterfly: 1 minute

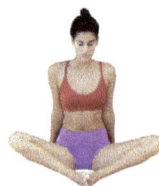

Side Stretch:
3–5 reps each side

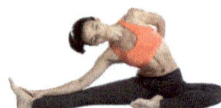

Knee to Chest: 3–5 reps

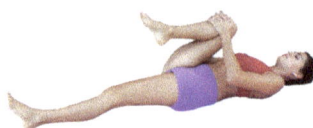

Supine Twist: 2–3 reps each side

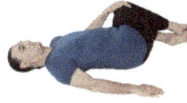

Bridge Version I (Basic Bridge): 3 reps

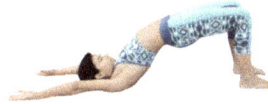

Bridge Version II (Open Bridge): 3 reps

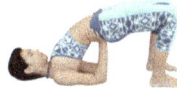

Snake Training I: 3–5 reps

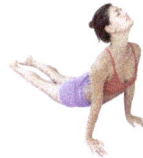

The Cat: 3–5 reps

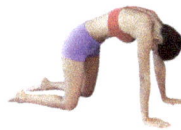

Four Keys

First Key: Abdominal to Intercostal: 3 rounds

Second Key: Intercostal to Chest: 3 rounds

Third Key: Chest to Upper Chest: 3 rounds

Fourth Key: Collarbone: 3 rounds

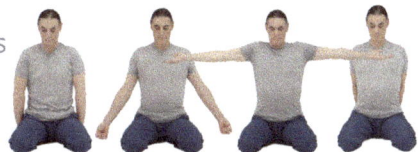

Exhaling from Top to Bottom

Stage 1: 2–3 rounds

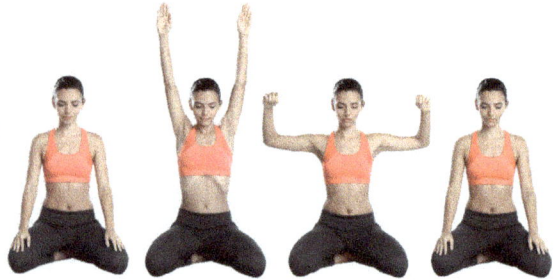

Rhythmic Breathing

(with the rhythms 4-4-4, 4-6-4, 4-8-4, 4-6-6): 5 rounds each, 1 **Purification Breathing** between each rhythm

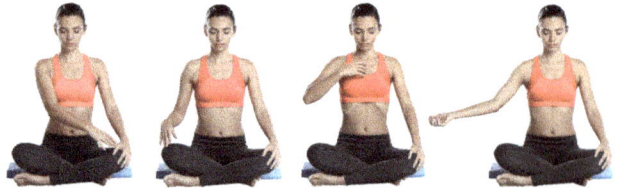

Coordinating the Four Phases

Coordinating Bridge (with pause): 3–5 rounds

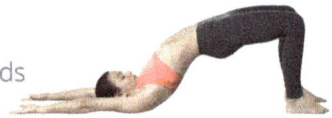

Complete Relaxation

2 minutes

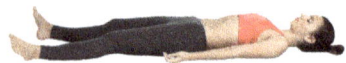

PASSIVE BALANCING AND CALMING: 15–18-MINUTE ROUTINE

Purification Breathing

3 rounds

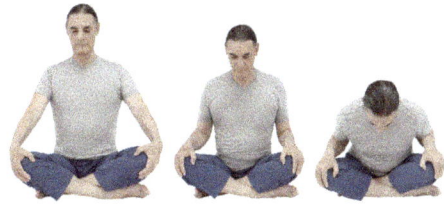

Abdominal Phase

Exercise 1 (Chin Tuck): 3 rounds

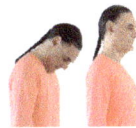

Exercise 2 (Shaping Bridge): 3 rounds

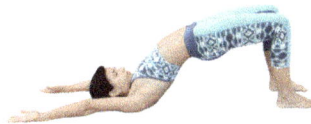

Exercise 3 (Open Bridge): 3 rounds

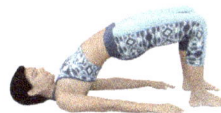

Relax, Open, and Discover

Supine Twist (experiencing opening at different levels): 3 minutes
Resting Dove (for abdominal and lateral dorsal expansion): 2 minutes

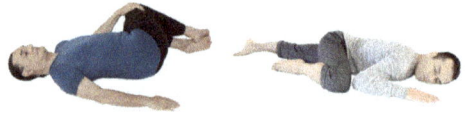

Dorsal Breathing

Exercise 1 (Knee-Hugging Squat):
1–2 minutes

or

Exercise 2 (Simplified Dorsal Training):
1–2 minutes

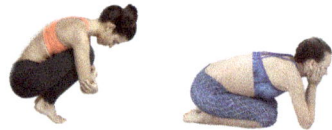

Thoracic Phase

Exercise 1 (Chest Opener, supported or unsupported): 2–3 minutes

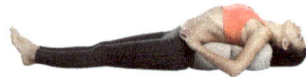

Exercise 2 (Active Upper Chest Opener): 3–5 rounds

or

Exercise 4 (Forward-Resting Chest Opener II): 3–5 rounds

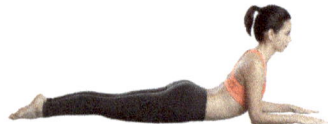

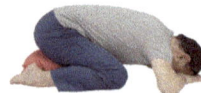

Rhythmic Breathing

(with the rhythms 4-4-4, 4-6-4, 4-8-4, 4-6-6): 5 rounds each, 1 **Purification Breathing** between each rhythm

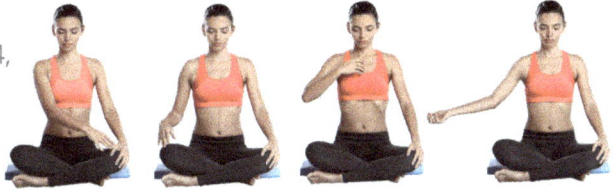

Natural Breathing

(with or without support): 2–3 minutes

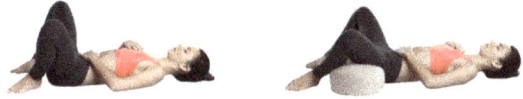

Complete Relaxation

2–3 minutes

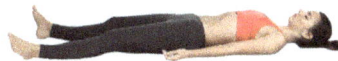

APPENDIX 3 |

HEALTH BENEFITS OF HARMONIOUS BREATHING

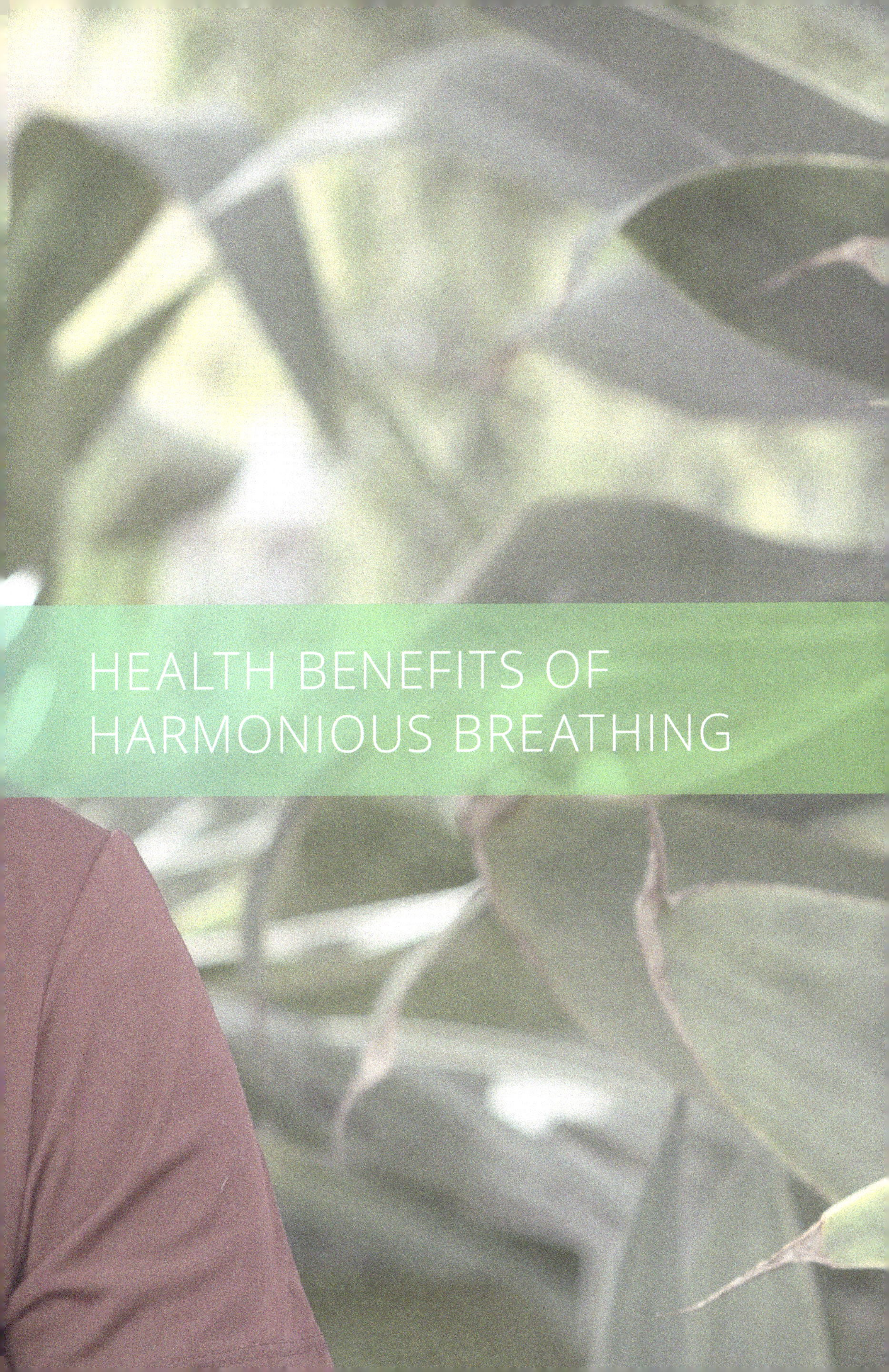

HEALTH BENEFITS OF HARMONIOUS BREATHING

THE POWER OF BREATH

When asked about the function of the respiratory system, most people answer that it supplies our bloodstream with oxygen and removes carbon dioxide from it. But this is a gross understatement. In fact, apart from serving as a base for all forms of speech, enabling the sense of smell, and aiding the processes of urination, defecation, and childbirth, breathing has several other important functions:[i]

1. Maintaining the correct pH: Since carbon dioxide generates acid in reaction with water, expelling it through the exhalation prevents acidosis, or abnormally low levels of pH. The pH of cerebrospinal fluid, in turn, affects neural functions – it can make you excited or depressed. An imbalance in acidity can also affect neuromuscular function.

2. Controlling blood pressure: The lungs help synthesize angiotensin II,[ii] a hormone responsible for increasing blood pressure. Several drugs used for treating hypertension decrease the production rate of angiotensin II. Evidence suggests that deep, regular breathing, with thorough inhalations and exhalations, effectively lowers blood pressure (discussed in more detail below).

3. Circulating blood and lymph: The pressure created between the thorax and abdomen promotes the flow of lymph and venous blood.

4. Filtering the blood: You have probably heard how dangerous blood clots are. You may not know, however, that the lungs filter smaller blood clots and actually dissolve them, preventing them from entering important arteries.

5. Exchanging gases: The most commonly recognized function of breathing. The process of inhaling and exhaling removes carbon dioxide from the blood and supplies oxygen, which is subsequently transported by the circulatory system to body cells so that they can release energy.

As you can see, respiration is deeply connected to several other organ systems, and an imbalance in breathing can affect us in many different ways.

THE THREE-PART RESPIRATORY SYSTEM

On an anatomical level, the respiratory system is composed of three parts: the upper respiratory tract, the lower respiratory tract, and the diaphragm.

The upper respiratory tract essentially consists of the nasal passages, the mouth, and the pharynx. The lower respiratory tract begins below the vocal folds, and includes the trachea, or windpipe, the bronchi, and the lungs. The lungs are spongy organs housing the respiratory tree, a vast network of increasingly fine airways ending with the alveoli, the tiny air sacs where gas exchange takes place.

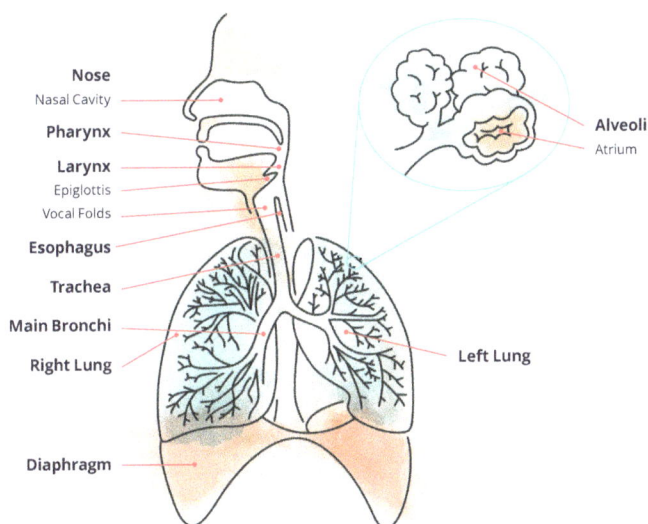

Nose
Nasal Cavity
Pharynx
Larynx
Epiglottis
Vocal Folds
Esophagus
Trachea
Main Bronchi
Right Lung
Diaphragm
Alveoli
Atrium
Left Lung

THE ROLE OF THE DIAPHRAGM

The lungs are highly elastic, largely passive organs; the process of contraction and expansion – inhalation and exhalation – that pulls air into the lungs is mainly driven by the movement of the diaphragm.

In the inhalation phase, the dome of the diaphragm flattens and lowers as it expands outward. This dropping of the diaphragm creates greater volume, and therefore less pressure, in the thoracic cavity. Air flows into the lungs to equalize the thoracic pressure with the atmospheric pressure. As the lungs expand, the external intercostal muscles come into play, lifting the rib cage and expanding it in three dimensions, front to back, in length, and out to the sides.

To accommodate the expansion of the lungs, the abdominal organs move downward and outward from the center. This is why when breathing properly it feels as if we are breathing "into the abdomen," while in fact the air is entering only the lungs.

The phase of exhalation starts when the main inspiratory muscles (diaphragm and external intercostal muscles) relax. The relaxation causes the diaphragm, attached to the spine by ligaments known as the crura, to ascend and narrow, and the ribs descend passively until the last bit of the exhalation - when the internal intercostal muscles come into play. At the very end of an exhalation where all breath is expelled, the abdominal muscles also become active.

In order to breathe in, we must flatten the dome-shaped diaphragm; to breathe out, we let it relax again. The diaphragm delivers oxygen to us a dozen times or more each minute, a half-billion times during an 80-year life. "We are completely dependent on the diaphragm," says Gabrielle Kardon, a biologist at the University of Utah. "But we take it for granted every moment we're breathing."

(Carl Zimmer, "Behind Each Breath, an Underappreciated Muscle")

Optimum movement of the diaphragm, and hence the organs, is crucial for good health because it stimulates blood flow and prevents stagnation and toxins from building up in the organs. In addition, the full expansion of the lungs leads to more effective and efficient oxygenation of the cells, tissues, and organs. Aside from the increase in volume, since three times as many blood vessels are present in the lower region of the lungs compared to the upper lung area, complete breathing with full activation of the diaphragm further boosts the respiratory exchange of oxygen and carbon dioxide and optimizes the oxygen-carbon dioxide balance.

The less freely the diaphragm moves, the less easily you breathe and the more anxious you feel.

(Jillian Pransky, "Restorative Yoga 101")

While carbon dioxide is a waste product, if the amount expelled with exhalations exceeds the amount produced in the body, a condition call hyperventilation can occur. Unless the body manages to compensate metabolically, blood pH rises, resulting in symptoms that can range from dizziness and tingling to headaches, fainting, and seizures.

Both in chronic upper chest breathing, where the diaphragm is not properly activated, and in shallow breathing triggered by situations of stress and anxiety, less oxygen is available and more carbon dioxide is expelled. When carbon dioxide levels drop, we experience increased feelings of anxiety, perpetuating the shallow breathing patterns. To compensate for the lower oxygen levels, red blood cell production increases, thickening the blood and making the heart beat faster and harder. This, in turn, raises blood pressure.

Inferior Breathing

Inhalation

Lungs and rib cage expand upward

Abdomen draws inward

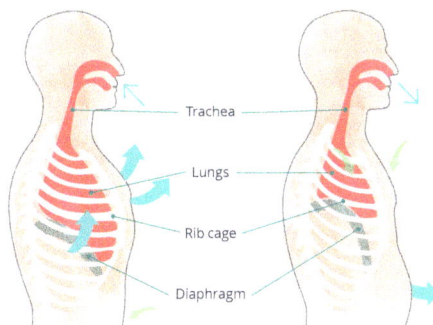

Trachea

Lungs

Rib cage

Diaphragm

Exhalation

Ribs collapse inward and downward

Downward movement in chest pushes abdomen down and belly out

Correct Breathing

Inhalation

Diaphragm contracts and moves downward, making space for the lungs to expand

External intercostal muscles contract for additional upward and outward expansion

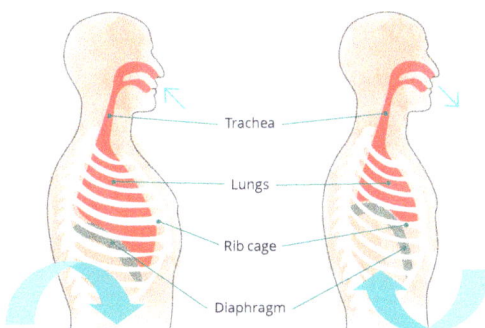

Trachea

Lungs

Rib cage

Diaphragm

Exhalation

Diaphragm relaxes and rises as rib cage descends, aided by internal intercostal muscles

Abdominal muscles contract and abdomen draws inward

The diaphragm muscle not only plays a role in respiration but also has many roles affecting the health of the body. It is important for posture, for proper organ function, and for the pelvis and floor of the mouth. It is important for the cervical spine and trigeminal system, as well as for the thoracic outlet. It is also of vital importance in the vascular and lymphatic systems. The diaphragm muscle should not be seen as a segment but as part of a body system.

(Bruno Bordoni and Emiliano Zanier, "Anatomic connections of the diaphragm: influence of respiration on the body system")

The central importance of the diaphragm in bringing oxygen in and carbon dioxide out of the lungs explains why complete breathing focuses on training this vital respiratory muscle.

WHY HEART RATE VARIABILITY MATTERS

Our breathing and heart rate are intrinsically linked and interdependent. Since our heart rate speeds up when we inhale and slows down when we exhale, the variation in the time gap between beats – referred to as heart rate variability or HRV – is closely related to the quality of our breathing.

It is known that HRV and respiration rate affect each other. [...] The heart and the respiratory system are irregular oscillators and the interaction is weak. If, however, respiration is guided, one of the oscillators becomes regular. If this pace is slow the synchronization dependence between the two oscillators increases and becomes stronger: slow respiration produces higher HRV amplitudes.

(Vickhoff et al., "Music structure determines heart rate variability of singers")

Studies have shown that slow respiration produces higher HRV amplitudes, and that an optimal level of HRV reflects healthy function and an inherent self-regulatory capacity, adaptability, or resilience. While too much instability is detrimental to efficient physiological functioning and energy utilization, too little variation indicates age-related system depletion, chronic stress, pathology, or inadequate functioning in various levels of self-regulatory control systems.

Neuroanatomic and brain imaging studies reveal breath-activated pathways to all major networks involved in emotion regulation, cognitive function, attention, perception, subjective awareness, and decision making. Specific breath practices have been shown to be beneficial in reducing symptoms of stress, anxiety, insomnia, posttraumatic stress disorder, obsessive-compulsive disorder, depression, attention deficit disorder, and schizophrenia.

(Brown et al., "Breathing Practices for Treatment of Psychiatric and Stress-Related Medical Conditions")

Recent findings on breathing techniques have led to the emergence of new treatments for stress and stress-related medical conditions, anxiety disorders, depression, posttraumatic stress disorder (PTSD), and attention-deficit disorder. The study cited above found that breathing practices can reduce aberrations in sympatho-vagal balance, stress response, emotion regulation, and neuroendocrine function, all of which are associated with these conditions.

Research increasingly recognizes the important role that practices such as breathwork, yoga, qigong, and tai chi can have in improving HRV and promoting balance between the sympathetic and parasympathetic nervous systems (associated with "fight-or-flight" and "rest-and-digest" responses, respectively). Specifically, these practices can stimulate the parasympathetic system and help overcome a dominance of fight-or-flight responses like stress and anxiety.

BREATHING AND BLOOD PRESSURE

Elevated blood pressure or hypertension is the leading cause of cardiovascular mortality. This medical condition is particularly dangerous since it doesn't necessarily produce any symptoms while damaging internal organs over an extended period of time. Patients are generally advised to exercise, lose weight, reduce sodium intake and, if necessary, take medication. As scientific research demonstrates, deep breathing, characterized by full, long inhalations and exhalations, can aid in lowering blood pressure, and in some situations can be as effective as a pill.

Since full, deep breathing can reduce stress,[iii] it can also reduce blood pressure.[iv] The normal breath rate is between 12 and 15 breaths a minute. Scientists have discovered that lowering this value to 10 by gradually prolonging the exhalation and keeping it at this level for at least 15 minutes can significantly reduce blood pressure, and the effect can last long after the session.[v] This kind of breathing exercise is therefore extremely useful for anyone suffering from hypertension.

LOWER HEART RATE AND STRESS REDUCTION

Stress is prevalent in modern life: while we no longer need to hunt for survival, we inherited from our ancestors the same biological mechanisms that allowed them to physically attack their prey with full force or make a run for it when in danger. Several factors influence our stress level, and sensitivity to it varies greatly from person to person. Even though we can't avoid situations that trigger a stress response, and conscious, direct control over stress is difficult to achieve, we can help ourselves indirectly by using breathing exercises such as the one described above (lowering the breath rate to 10 full respirations a minute by gradually making the exhalations longer).

We can directly experience the benefits of this technique by measuring our heart rate just after a stressful event and after a breathing exercise. The measurement itself can be done easily with just a smartphone and a free app. Usually, it's enough to put a finger on the lens of the camera; the app then turns on the flashlight and measures variations in blood flow in the finger over time. Heart rate measurements taken in this way are fairly accurate.

If we compare heart rate under stress and after several full, long breaths, we can easily notice (and measure, as described above) the difference. Heart rate is an accurate measure of stress: it's virtually impossible to be under stress and maintain a normal heart rate. As you'll notice, a breathing exercise can be of enormous help in regaining a calm state of mind – something that is not easy to achieve by thinking alone.[vi]

How does it actually work? Recent scientific research at Stanford University demonstrated that certain breathing-related nerves in the brain are directly connected to the arousal center of the brain. That means breathing is related to overall brain activity.[vii]

A CURE FOR DEPRESSION

Even though there is not enough evidence to suggest that depression can be completely cured with breathing exercises alone, it is quite possible that they can improve the condition considerably. Recent research by scientists from the University of Pennsylvania demonstrated that patients who were resistant to antidepressant medication – in other words, "incurable" by conventional means – responded favorably to a set of yoga and breathing exercises performed over a period of two months.

As the study was conducted by psychiatrists rather than neuroscientists, in this case the researchers focused on the results rather than the underlying mechanisms, trying to test an alternative therapy for those for whom conventional medication is ineffective. The symptoms of depression are a prolonged sense of sadness, a pessimistic attitude, lowered self-esteem, general loss of interest in life and activities, and often insomnia and a loss of appetite. The results of the study are promising: the tested group improved by 10.27 points on the Hamilton Rating Scale for Depression, whereas the control group showed no signs of improvement.[viii] The result of the study gives hope to all those who find traditional treatment for depression ineffective. Moreover, when applied correctly, yoga and breathing exercises are relatively safe and have no negative side effects.

POSTURE AND BREATHING

For every movement we make and in every position we pause, the breath is, in one way or another, affected by that action or position.

It is generally accepted that poor posture contributes to the dysfunctional breathing patterns of fragmented and shallow breathing. Many occupations in modern life require long hours of sitting, particularly those in front of a computer screen, which encourage jaw to shoot forward, the shoulders to round, and the back to slouch. Prolonged smartphone usage has the same impact on posture.[ix] In general, these postural characteristics block the possibility of breathing properly.

Conversely, since posture and breathing go hand in hand, by learning how to breathe fully, smoothly, and fluidly, such as in Harmonious Breathing, we will automatically improve our posture.

CURRENT AND FUTURE RESEARCH

Researchers from many parts of the world are conducting interesting studies on the positive influence of breathing exercises on various areas of life, and more news on the subject is being published just about every day.

Visit www.harmoniousbreathing.com for updates on latest research findings.

---

[i] Kenneth S. Saladin, *Human Anatomy*, 654.

[ii] *Wikipedia's* entry on angiotensin II ("ACE is a target of ACE inhibitor drugs, which decrease the rate of angiotensin II production. Angiotensin II increases blood pressure by stimulating the Gq protein...").

[iii] Crystal Goh, "Brain's Remote Control." ("...slow, steady breathing activates the calming part of our nervous system, and slows our heart rate, reducing feelings of anxiety and stress.")

[iv] Naomi D. L. Fisher, "Stress raising blood pressure?"

[v] Ibid. "There is only one non-drug treatment approved for hypertension by the FDA – a device called RESPeRATE. It uses musical tones to guide deep abdominal breathing. Its goal is to reduce the number of breaths to under 10 per minute, and to prolong each exhalation. Clinical trials have shown that daily RESPeRATE use lowered blood pressure, sometimes as much as a blood pressure pill would have. This lowering effect also lasted long after each session."

[vi] Alice Park, "Fastest Way to Calm Down."

[vii] Christina Zelano et al., "Nasal Respiration."

[viii] Marna S. Barrett, et al., "Yogic Breathing."

[ix] Sang In Jung, et al., "The effect of smartphone usage time."

GLOSSARY

abdominal breathing. A term used in this book to indicate the "below-first" phase of the inhalation in **complete breathing**. The word abdominal refers to the sensation of the breath expanding into the abdomen, although in actuality the air is expanding in the lungs only. As the lungs fill and the diaphragm moves down, the abdomen expands, but when done correctly this should occur without bloating or overinflating. During exhalation, from the top down, the diaphragm moves upward again, causing the abdomen to naturally deflate.

Ayurveda. The traditional medical system of India, generally considered to have originated some five thousand years ago. Numerous parallels exist between Ayurveda and **Tibetan medicine**, notably the identification of three humors, energies, or *doshas* (a Sanskrit term that literally means "fault" or "deficiency") and the concept that their balance or imbalance determines good or poor health. Ayurveda applies numerous modalities of treatment, ranging from the use of herbal and mineral substances to diet and massage.

Chögyal Namkhai Norbu. Born in Eastern Tibet in 1938, Chögyal Namkhai Norbu is an internationally known **Dzogchen** master and author as well as an eminent scholar of the history and culture of Tibet. In the 1960s, he was invited to Italy as a professor of Tibetology, where about a decade later he began to give instructions to a growing following of Western students on Yantra Yoga and Dzogchen, the Total Perfection teaching, until then unknown outside of Tibet. He inspired the founding of the International Dzogchen Community, created to encourage the teaching and practice of the Dzogchen point of view and meditation methods, and travels worldwide giving teachings and speaking at international conferences. A prolific author of books on Dzogchen, Yantra Yoga, and Tibetan history, medicine, and culture, he founded ASIA and the Shang Shung Institute (now the Shang Shung Foundation), two nonprofit organizations dedicated to supporting the Tibetan people and preserving Tibetan culture.

complete breathing. An ideal and complete respiratory pattern in which both inhalation and exhalation fluidly combine an abdominal, an intercostal, and a thoracic phase. In **Harmonious Breathing**, the third phase is further subdivided into a chest phase and an upper chest phase, making four in all. Complete breathing is a fundamental quality of breathing in **Yantra Yoga** and Harmonious Breathing. It promotes health and well-being and is the key to a positive, relaxed state of mind, sound sleep, good digestion, and stabilized blood pressure, among other benefits. Inhaling through the nostrils, the lungs are gradually filled from the bottom to the top, like a vase being filled with water. Exhaling through the nostrils, the top of the lungs is emptied first and the lower part of the lungs last. The ideal shape of the inhalation and the exhalation can be compared a grain of barley, starting slowly, opening to a stronger flow, and tapering off to a smooth, gradual end. The mind is present, relaxed but alert and focused on the unified flow of breathing and movement.

diaphragmatic breathing. In this book, the term diaphragmatic breathing is generally used in connection with **abdominal breathing** to indicate the active involvement of the diaphragm in below-first inhalation. Yoga expert David H. Coulter makes a distinction between what he calls abdomino-diaphragmatic breathing, essentially connoting what we refer to here as the abdominal phase, and thoraco-diaphragmatic breathing, where the emphasis is more on the rib cage.

dorsal breathing. Rather than constituting a separate phase of **complete breathing**, dorsal breathing refers to a quality that can augment each of the main phases. Expanding the dorsal breathing capacity is especially beneficial for people who have a tight, blocked diaphragm and a habit of shallow breathing.

Dzogchen. The Tibetan word Dzogchen means "total" (*chen*) "perfection" (*dzog*), the real condition of each individual. It refers to the self-perfected state, the potentiality of our real nature. The method for acquiring knowledge of Dzogchen and discovering our real condition is called Dzogchen teaching. It is not a philosophical theory created by intellectual analysis but rather a direct experience. Knowledge of Dzogchen goes back to ancient times. Dzogchen practitioners are found in nearly every school of Tibetan Buddhism as well as in Bön. The teaching was first introduced in the West by **Chögyal Namkhai Norbu**. For more information, visit www.dzogchen.net.

Harmonious Breathing. Developed by Fabio Andrico, Harmonious Breathing is a simple and effective method that teaches us experientially how to rediscover a fluid, complete respiration pattern and integrate it in our lives. It calms the mind, reduces tension in the body, and improves both physiological and cerebral functions. Conscious, mindful breathing is used in many relaxation methods, and is central to practices such as yoga. Its contribution to health and harmony has been known in Eastern cultures for many centuries, and is now widely recognized in the West as well. Drawing on the knowledge that the position of the body influences the flow of the breath, in Harmonious Breathing a wide range of positions are used to explore how each can affect the movement of the breath within the body. To be effective, the positions are combined with presence, awareness, and an understanding of the principles of complete breathing. Harmonious Breathing fully engages all parts of the body involved in the breathing process, from the diaphragm to the abdominal, intercostal, and back muscles. It gently exercises these muscles, flushes out the lymphatic system, and improves the balance of oxygen and carbon dioxide throughout the body. Visit www.harmoniousbreathing.com for more information and online classes.

heart rate variability (HRV). The variation in the time interval between heartbeats. Since our heart rate speeds up when we inhale and slows down when we exhale, HRV is closely related to the quality of our breathing. When heart rate variability and breathing rhythms are synchronized, our sympathetic and parasympathetic functions are balanced and a synergy is produced between the autonomic and somatic branches of the central nervous system. Studies have shown that slow respiration produces higher HRV amplitudes, and that an optimal level of HRV reflects healthy function and an inherent self-regulatory capacity, adaptability, or resilience.

hyperventilation. When the amount of carbon dioxide expelled with exhalations exceeds the amount produced in the body, a condition call hyperventilation can occur (also called overbreathing). Unless the body manages to compensate metabolically, blood pH rises, resulting in symptoms that can range from dizziness and tingling to headaches, fainting, and seizures. Overdoing any kind of exercise can cause the volume of carbon dioxide ventilated to exceed the body's production of it, and this, in turn, leads to hyperventilation. This is why it is important to always pace ourselves when exercising. Additionally, breathing through the nostrils, which is always implied in Harmonious Breathing, prevents any risks of hyperventilation.

intercostal breathing. In the intercostal phase, the second of the three main phases in **complete breathing**, the air expands into the middle part of the lungs at the level of the mid-lower ribcage. During an inhalation, the downward motion of the diaphragm and the contraction of the intercostal muscles pull the rib cage both upward and outward, creating more space in the chest cavity. The opposite happens during an exhalation.

prana. Sanskrit term referring to the essence of life, our energy, power, life force. Some sources consider it to be synonymous with the breath itself. Related to the air element, it is equally fundamental in **Traditional Tibetan Medicine**, where it is called *lung*. In Traditional Chinese Medicine, *qi* is a similar principle, and many other ancient cultures link the force of life directly to the breath.

tidal volume. The volume of air inhaled and exhaled in one cycle during normal breathing at rest. In that sense, it represents the most average range of an individual's lung volume. When we inhale within our tidal volume, the action of the inspiratory muscles is moderate; usually only the diaphragm is involved. Pulmonary elasticity is stretched only slightly. Breathing out, the expiratory muscles are relaxed and inactive; the lungs return to their original shape mainly as a result of pulmonary elasticity.

Traditional Tibetan Medicine (TTM). A practice of medicine that evolved over several thousand years, dating back to the pre-Buddhist Bön era in Tibet. Over time, it absorbed influences from Ayurveda, traditional Chinese, Byzantine, and Persian medicine, as well as from nearby countries like Nepal. Tibetan traditional medicine centers on the principle that the functioning of the human body is determined by the interaction of the three humors or energies: wind, bile, and phlegm. It views illnesses as the result of imbalances of the humors, among other factors, as a consequence of emotions such as ignorance, greed, and anger. Modes of treatment range from dietary and behavioral changes, including the introduction of appropriate physical exercise such as **Yantra Yoga**, to the administration of medicines composed of natural substances and the application of external therapies.

vagus nerve. The longest cranial nerve, also known as the "wandering nerve" (*vagus* literally means "wandering"). Its multiple branches diverge from the cerebellum and brainstem and wander to the lowest reaches of the abdomen, touching the heart and most major organs along the way. In the early twentieth century, German physiologist Otto Loewi discovered that stimulating the vagus nerve causes a reduction in heart rate by triggering the release of a substance later identified as acetylcholine. This substance is like a tranquilizer that we can activate simply by taking a few deep breaths with long exhales, creating a state of inner calm while taming our inflammatory reflex. The vagus nerve is the central component of the parasympathetic nervous system, regulator of the "rest-and-digest" or "tend-and-befriend" responses. Conversely, the sympathetic nervous system drives the "fight-or-flight" response. Healthy vagal tone is indicated by a slight increase of heart rate on inhalations and a decrease of heart rate on exhalations, the hallmark of greater **heart rate variability**. The improved tone of the diaphragm muscle developed in complete breathing gently activates our inner organs and hence stimulates the vagus nerve, which explains its many beneficial effects.

Yantra Yoga. An ancient Tibetan practice first introduced to the West in the 1970s by **Dzogchen** master **Chögyal Namkhai Norbu**. Yantra Yoga promotes optimal health, relaxation, and meditation through the coordination of breath and movement. Consisting of three groups of preliminary exercises, five series of Yantra movements, and several *pranayama* (breathing) exercises, it is taught all over the world by a growing number of accredited instructors. It features unique sequences of movement that experientially teach us how to improve and expand our breathing capacity, consequently bringing benefits to multiple levels of our being, from body to mind and energy. For more information, visit www.yantrayoga.org.

BIBLIOGRAPHY

Anyen Rinpoche and Allison Choying Zangmo. *The Tibetan Yoga of Breath: Breathing Exercises for Healing the Body and Cultivating Wisdom*. Boston and London: Shambhala, 2013.

Barrett, Marna S., Andrew J. Cucchiara, Nalaka S. Gooneratne, Michael E. Thase, et al., "Yogic Breathing Helps Fight Major Depression, Penn Study Shows," *Penn Medicine News*, November 22, 2016, https://www.pennmedicine.org/news/news-releases/2016/november/yogic-breathing-helps-fight-ma.

Bordoni, Bruno, and Emiliano Zanier. "Anatomic connections of the diaphragm: influence of respiration on the body system." *Journal of Multidisciplinary Healthcare* no. 6 (2013), 281–291. doi: 10.2147/JMDH.S45443.

Brown, Richard P., Patricia L. Gerbarg, Fred Muench. "Breathing Practices for Treatment of Psychiatric and Stress-Related Medical Conditions." *Psychiatric Clinics of North America* 36, no. 1 (2013), 121–140. doi: 10.1016/j.psc.2013.01.001.

Calais-Germain, Blandine. *Anatomy of Breathing*. Seattle: Eastland Press, 2006.

Chögyal Namkhai Norbu. *Birth, Life and Death*. Translated by Elio Guarisco. Arcidosso: Shang Shung Publications, 2008.

———. *Rainbow Body: The Life and Realization of Togden Ugyen Tendzin*. Arcidosso: Shang Shung Edizioni, 2010.

———. *Yantra Yoga: The Tibetan Yoga of Movement*. Translated by Adriano Clemente. Ithaca: Snow Lion Publications, 2008.

Chögyal Namkhai Norbu and Fabio Andrico, *Tibetan Yoga of Movement: The Art and Practice of Yantra Yoga*. Arcidosso: Shang Shung Publications, Berkeley: North Atlantic Books, 2013.

Coulter, H. David. *Anatomy of Hatha Yoga: A Manual for Students, Teachers, and Practitioners*. Honesdale: Body and Breath, 2001.

Fisher, Naomi D. L. "Stress raising your blood pressure? Take a deep breath." *Harvard Health* (blog), http://www.health.harvard.edu/blog/stress-raising-your-blood-pressure-take-a-deep-breath-201602159168.

Goh, Crystal. "Your Breath Is Your Brain's Remote Control." *Mindful*, February 16, 2017, https://www.mindful.org/breath-brains-remote-control/.

Guarisco, Elio, and Phuntsog Wangmo. *Healing with Yantra Yoga: From Tibetan Medicine to the Subtle Body*. With excerpts from talks by Chögyal Namkhai Norbu. Arcidosso: Shang Shung Publications, 2016.

Iyengar, B.K.S., with John J. Evans and Douglas Abrams. *Light on Life: The Yoga Journey to Wholeness, Inner Peace, and Ultimate Freedom*. Reprint ed. New York: Rodale Books, 2006.

Kaminoff, Leslie. *Yoga Anatomy*. 2nd ed. Champaign: Human Kinetics, 2012.

McCraty, Rollin, and Fred Shaffer. "Heart Rate Variability: New Perspectives on Physiological Mechanisms, Assessment of Self-regulatory Capacity, and Health Risk." *Global Advances in Health and Medicine* no. 4 (1): 46–61 (2015). doi: 10.7453/gahmj.2014.073.

Park, Alice. "This Is the Fastest Way to Calm Down." *Time*, March 30, 2017, http://time.com/4718723/deep-breathing-meditation-calm-anxiety/.

Pransky, Jillian. "Restorative Yoga 101: How to Release Chronic Psoas Tension for Deeper Relaxation." *Yoga Journal*, September 5, 2017, https://www.yogajournal.com/yoga-101/restorative-yoga-101-how-to-release-chronic-psoas-tension-for-deeper-relaxation.

Saladin, Kenneth S. *Human Anatomy*. New York: McGraw Hill, 2007.

Sang In Jung, Na Kyung Lee, Kyung Woo Kang, Kyoung Kim, and Do Youn Lee. "The effect of smartphone usage time on posture and respiratory function." *Journal of Physical Therapy Science* 28, no. 1 (2016), 186–189. doi:10.1589/jpts.28.186.

Telles, Shirley, Nilkamal Singh, Meesha Joshi, and Acharya Balkrishna. "Post traumatic stress symptoms and heart rate variability in Bihar flood survivors following yoga: a randomized controlled study." *BMC Psychiatry* 10:18 (2010). https://bmcpsychiatry.biomedcentral.com/articles/10.1186/1471-244X-10-18.

Vickhoff, Björn, Helge Malmgren, Rickard Åström, Gunnar Nyberg, Seth-Reino Ekström, Mathias Engwall, Johan Snygg, Michael Nilsson, and Rebecka Jörnsten. "Music structure determines heart rate variability of singers." *Frontiers in Psychology* no. 4: 334. doi:10.3389/fpsyg.2013.00334.

Zelano, Christina, Heidi Jiang, Guangyu Zhou, Nikita Arora, Stephan Schuele, Joshua Rosenow, and Jay A. Gottfried, "Nasal Respiration Entrains Human Limbic Oscillations and Modulates Cognitive Function." *Journal of Neuroscience,* December 7, 2016, 36 (49) 12448-12467. doi:10.1523/JNEUROSCI.2586-16.

Zimmer, Carl. "Behind Each Breath, an Underappreciated Muscle." *New York Times*, April 2, 2015.

INDEX OF EXERCISES BY LEVEL

CORE EXERCISES

CORE EXERCISES

WARM-UPS

WARM-UPS

ABOUT THE AUTHOR

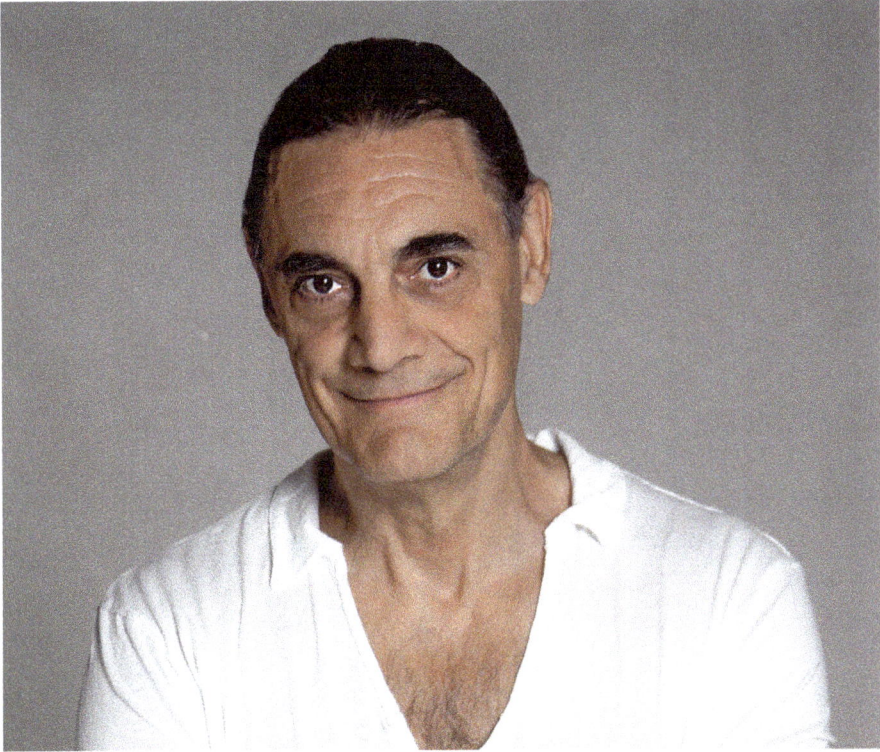

Born and raised in Italy, Fabio Andrico is an internationally recognized expert on Yantra Yoga. He is one of the closest students of Chögyal Namkhai Norbu, the great Tibetan master who introduced Dzogchen and Yantra Yoga to the West in the early 1970s. Andrico, who initially studied Hatha Yoga in India and graduated in Oriental studies at University of Naples "L'Orientale," has been learning, practicing, teaching, and writing about Yantra Yoga since the late 1970s. He regularly conducts courses, workshops, and teacher trainings around the world, at venues including Kripalu, Esalen, and Yoga Tree in the USA and Yoga Federation in Russia. Drawing on decades of experience, he developed Harmonious Breathing, a comprehensive method for learning how to breathe smoothly and consciously for health and well-being. He teaches it internationally with the support of a growing team of accredited instructors. Andrico has appeared in videos such as *BreAthe*, *The Eight Movements of Yantra Yoga*, and *Tibetan Yoga of Movement, Levels 1 and 2*, and also collaborated on the book *Yantra Yoga: The Tibetan Yoga of Movement*.

www.ingramcontent.com/pod-product-compliance
Lightning Source LLC
Chambersburg PA
CBHW041017280326
41926CB00094B/4658